Best of Five MCQs for the Endocrinology and Diabetes SCE

Best of Five MCQs for the Endocrinology and Diabetes SCE

Edited by

Dr Atul Kalhan
FRCP MD (Cardiff University) MD (Delhi University) MRCPE

Consultant Physician/Diabetes & Endocrinology,
Cardiff & Vale University Healthboard, Cardiff, UK

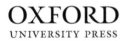

OXFORD
UNIVERSITY PRESS

OXFORD
UNIVERSITY PRESS

Great Clarendon Street, Oxford, OX2 6DP,
United Kingdom

Oxford University Press is a department of the University of Oxford.
It furthers the University's objective of excellence in research, scholarship,
and education by publishing worldwide. Oxford is a registered trade mark of
Oxford University Press in the UK and in certain other countries

Published in the United States of America by Oxford University Press
198 Madison Avenue, New York, NY 10016, United States of America

British Library Cataloguing in Publication Data
Data available

Library of Congress Control Number: 2014954175

ISBN 978–0–19–872933–4

FOREWORD

The clinical practice of diabetes and endocrinology has a breadth and a depth unrivalled in contemporary medicine. The recognition that both the vascular endothelium and the adipocyte should be considered as endocrine organs in their own right, the exponential increase in the prevalence of type 2 diabetes, obesity, and the metabolic syndrome, with their attendant clinical sequelae, together with the more traditional endocrine disorders emphasizes the point. The broad range of scientific disciplines range from molecular genetics through to medical biochemistry. This breadth and depth confers a logistical challenge for the provision of appropriate comprehensive clinical training for future specialists in the field.

This book is an excellent adjunct to the traditional text books. It is a comprehensive test of the reader's understanding of basic principles and is suitable for trainees at all levels. It is well written—clear and authoritative in style and very clinically orientated. It is translational in nature, i.e. it links basic science to clinical practice in a very innovative and relevant manner.

The authors are established experts in their field and are of a generation where their own training programmes are a not too-distant memory. This book deserves to be widely read. I shall be strongly recommending it to all trainees in diabetes and endocrinology.

Dr Alan Rees BSc, MD, FRCP
Consultant Physician in Diabetes, Endocrinology and Clinical Lipidology

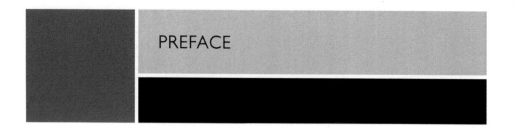

PREFACE

About a year and a half ago, huddled in one of the conference halls of annual diabetes UK meeting at Manchester, me and my fellow Diabetes & Endocrinology colleagues wondered about a lack of written resource for specialty certificate exam (SCE) which still was in its early years since inception. It was a more arduous task than we had anticipated and at one stage almost failed to take off, with the initial enthusiasm fading rapidly faced with the practical aspects of the complex task in hand. Only in the late winter of 2013 when the sun was making its customary fleeting guest appearances, I took it on myself (with able support from my colleagues) to burn midnight oil and give shape to this dream.

This book contains more than 300 best of five multiple choice questions with explanatory answers and up-to-date references/guidelines; it is an attempt to provide Diabetes & Endocrinology trainees with real life based clinical scenarios which will help them with the SCE exam besides bridging any gap in knowledge.

I am thankful to Oxford University press especially Geraldine and Fiona for patiently guiding me through the early phases of getting the correct format to the written text. I wish to express my gratitude to Gautam, Vinay, and Rao for taking the ownership of individual chapters and keeping spirits high. Lastly, I am indebted by the patience shown and constant encouragement provided by my wife Anu, who remained a pillar of support and took care of little ones while I was glued to my laptop writing/editing the text.

Atul

Dr Atul Kalhan
FRCP (Edinburgh) MD (Cardiff University) MD (Delhi University) MRCPE
Consultant Diabetes & Endocrinology/Physician
Cardiff & Vale University healthboard

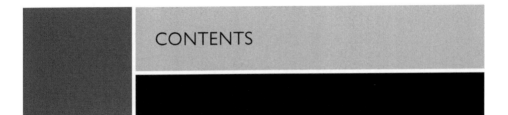

CONTENTS

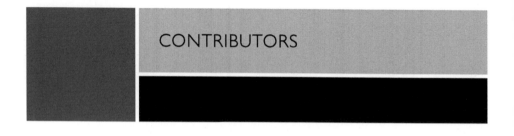
CONTRIBUTORS

Dr Atul Kalhan Consultant Physician/Diabetes & Endocrinology, Cardiff & Vale University Healthboard, Cardiff, UK

All Chapters

Dr Vinay Eligar Specialist Registrar, Cardiff & Vale University Healthboard, Cardiff, UK
Chapter 1 Pituitary gland and hypothalamus; Chapter 5 Reproductive endocrinology

Dr Gautam Das Consultant Diabetes & Endocrinology, Prince Charles Hospital, Merthyr Tydfil, UK
Chapter 2 Thyroid gland

Dr LNR Bondugulapati Locum Consultant (Diab & Endo), University Hospital of Wales, Cardiff UK
Chapter 3 Parathyroid gland and bone disease

ABBREVIATIONS

1° HPT	primary hyperparathyroidism
11β-HSD2	11β-hydroxy steroid dehydrogenase 2
17-OHP	17- hydroxy progesterone
2° HPT	secondary hyperparathyroidism
3β-HSD	3β-hydroxy steroid dehydrogenase
ACE	angiotensin-converting enzyme
ACR	albumin creatinine ratio
ACTH	adrenocorticotropic hormone
ADH	anti-diuretic hormone
AF	atrial fibrillation
AGHDA	assessment of growth hormone deficiency in adults
AIH	amiodarone-induced hypothyroidism
AIP	aryl hydrocarbon receptor-interacting protein
AIS	androgen insensitivity syndrome
AIT	amiodarone-induced thyrotoxicosis
ALP	alkaline phosphatase
ALT	alanine transaminase
AMH	anti-Müllerian hormone
Anti-TPO	anti-thyroid peroxidase
APA	aldosterone-producing adenoma
APCED	autoimmune polyendocrinopathy-candidiasis-ectodermal dystrophy
APS1	autoimmune polyglandular syndrome type I
ARR	aldosterone-to-renin ratio
BIPSS	bilateral inferior petrosal sinus sampling
CAH	congenital adrenal hyperplasia
CAS	clinical activity score
CaSR	calcium sensing receptor
CBG	corticosteroid-binding globulin
CD	constitutional delay
CKD	chronic kidney disease
CRH	corticotropin-releasing hormone
CRP	C-reactive protein

CBG	cortisol-binding globulin
DDAVP	desmopressin acetate
DHEA	dehydroepiandrosterone
DI	diabetes insipidus
DIO2	iodothyronine deiodinase Type 2
DM	diabetes mellitus
DMPA	depot medroxy progesterone
DOC	deoxycorticosterone
DPP4	dipeptidyl peptidase inhibitors 4
eGFR	estimated glomerular filtration rate
FFA	free fatty acid
FHH	familial hypocalciuric hypercalcaemia
FIPA	familial isolated pituitary adenomas
FNAC	fine needle aspiration cytology
FSH	follicle-stimulating hormone
FSHoma	FSH-secreting pituitary adenoma
FT4	free thyroxine
GAD	anti-glutamic acid decarboxylase
GC	glucocorticoids
GCS	Glasgow coma score
GD	Graves' disease
GDM	gestational diabetes
GH	growth hormone
GHD	growth hormone deficiency
GHRH	growth hormone releasing hormone
GLP-1	glucagon-like peptide
GnRH	gonadotropin-releasing hormone
GO	Graves' orbitopathy
GRA	glucocorticoid remedial hyperaldosteronism
H&E	haematoxylin and eosin
hCG	human chorionic gonadotropin
HDL	high-density lipoprotein
HLA	human leukocyte antigen
HNF	hepatocyte nuclear factor
HPA	hypothalamic–pituitary–adrenal
HPG	hypothalmo–pituitary–gonadal
hPL	human placental lactogen
HPLC	high pressure liquid chromatography
HRT	hormone replacement therapy
HU	Hounsfield units

IA-2	islet antigen 2
ICA	islet cell antigen
ICSI	intra-cytoplasmic sperm injection
IGFBP	insulin-like growth factor-binding protein
IHA	idiopathic hyperaldosteronism
IHD	ischaemic heart disease
ITT	insulin tolerance test
IVF	in vitro fertilization
LDDST	low dose dexamethasone suppression test
LDL	low-density lipoprotein
LH	luteinizing hormone
MDT	multidisciplinary team
MEN	multiple endocrine neoplasia
MODY	maturity onset diabetes of the young
MR	mineralocorticoid receptors
MTC	medullary thyroid cancer
NAFLD	non-alcoholic fatty liver disease
NCCAH	non-classic congenital adrenal hyperplasia
NFPA	non-functioning pituitary adenoma
NTIS	non-thyroidal illness syndrome
OCP	oral contraceptive pills
OGTT	oral glucose tolerance test
P450 scc	P450 side chain cleavage enzyme
PA	primary hyperaldosteronism
PCOS	polycystic ovarian syndrome
PGL	paraganglioma
PH	phaeochromocytoma
PHP	pseudohypoparathyroidism
PI	pituitary incidentaloma
PNMT	4-phenyethanolamine-N-methyltransferase
POMC	pro-opio-melano-corticotropin
PPNAD	primary pigmented nodular adrenocortical disease
PPT	post-partum thyroiditis
PRA	plasma renin activity
PRL	prolactin
PSA	prostate specific antigen
PTH	parathyroid hormone
PTHrP	PTH-related protein
PTU	propylthiouracil
RAI	radioactive iodine

RAIA	radioactive iodine ablation
RAIU	radioactive iodine uptake
RANK	receptor activator of nuclear factor kappa
RET	rearranged during transfection
SES	sick euthyroid syndrome
SGLT2	sodium-glucose co-transporter 2
SHBG	sex hormone-binding globulin
SIADH	syndrome of inappropriate antidiuretic hormone
SSTR	somatostatin receptor subtypes
TBG	thyroxine-binding globulin
TBPA	thyroxine-binding pre-albumin
TFT	thyroid function test
Tg	thyroglobulin
TRAB	TSH receptor antibodies
TRH	thyrotropin-releasing hormone
TSH	thyrotropin-stimulating hormone
TSHoma	TSH-secreting adenoma
TSH-R	TSH receptor
UFC	urinary free cortisol
VDDR	vitamin D-resistant rickets
VHL	Von Hippel–Lindau
VLCFA	very long chain fatty acids

PITUITARY GLAND AND HYPOTHALAMUS

QUESTIONS

1. Anterior pituitary cells are classified according to their staining properties and by their specific secretory products, which can be identified by immunocytochemical and electron microscopic techniques.

   Which one of the following is the most abundant cell population of the anterior pituitary gland?

   A. Corticotrophs
   B. Gonadotrophs
   C. Lactotrophs
   D. Somatotrophs
   E. Thyrotrophs

2. Anterior pituitary cells were originally classified based on their staining properties as: chromophil cells, which have staining property, and chromophobe cells, which do not stain very well in standard haematoxylin and eosin (H&E) preparations. The chromophil cells are subdivided into acidophil and basophil staining cells.

   Which one of the following anterior pituitary cell lines is acidophilic on H&E staining?

   A. β-endorphin secreting cells
   B. Corticotrophs
   C. Gonadotrophs
   D. Lactotrophs
   E. Thyrotrophs

3. **The secretion of adrenocorticotropic hormone (ACTH) follows a circadian rhythm with peak levels seen from 6 a.m. to 9 a.m., while the nadir is seen around 11 p.m. to 2 a.m.**

    ACTH release is under the influence of various pituitary and non-pituitary hormones.

    Which one of the following hormones is associated with a decreased ACTH release?
    A. Catecholamine
    B. Corticotropin-releasing hormone (CRH)
    C. Endocannabinoids
    D. Ghrelin
    E. Vasoactive intestinal peptide

4. **Growth hormone (GH) is secreted in a pulsatile manner, with around 5–10 pulses seen in a period of 24 hours. Women have higher mean GH levels compared with men.**

    Which one of the following factors/conditions is associated with an increased GH secretion?
    A. Ageing
    B. Increased BMI
    C. Lack of exercise
    D. Lack of sleep
    E. Type I diabetes mellitus

5. **Ghrelin, an important GH secretogogue, circulates mostly as the des-octanoylated form bound to a subfraction of high-density lipoprotein (HDL) particle.**

    Which one of the following is a biological action of ghrelin during normal physiological states?
    A. Decreased feeding
    B. Decreased utilization of metabolic substrates
    C. Increased gastric emptying
    D. Inhibition of GH secretion
    E. Inhibition of insulin secretion

6. **Vasopressin (antidiuretic hormone) is a nine-amino acid polypeptide that is synthesized in the hypothalamus and stored in the posterior pituitary. It acts as an important regulator of fluid and electrolyte balance.**

    Which one of the following is a known biological effect of vasopressin?
    A. Decreased ACTH secretion
    B. Decreased glycogenolysis
    C. Increased platelet adhesion
    D. Increased water reabsorption from proximal nephron
    E. Inhibition of smooth muscle contraction

7. Vasopressin secreted from the posterior pituitary gland has osmo- and baro-regulatory functions.

   Which one of the following factors is associated with a decreased vasopressin release from the posterior pituitary gland?
   A. Germinoma
   B. Head injury
   C. Increasing age
   D. Low blood pressure
   E. Lower respiratory infection

8. Oxytocin is a nine-amino acid polypeptide secreted from the posterior pituitary with most of its known or postulated physiological effects related to reproductive function in mammals.

   All of the following are known (or postulated) physiological actions of oxytocin except?
   A. Essential role in lactation
   B. Facilitation of birth
   C. Neurotransmitter
   D. Increased uterine contractions
   E. Social recognition and bonding

9. There are five major somatostatin receptor subtypes (SSTR 1–5) expressed in various organs in the body.

   Which one of the following combinations of subtypes of SSTRs is most commonly expressed in GH-secreting pituitary adenomas?
   A. SSTR-1 and SSTR-2
   B. SSTR-1 and SSTR-5
   C. SSTR-2 and SSTR-5
   D. SSTR-3 and SSTR-4
   E. SSTR-4 and SSTR-5

10. A 33-year-old woman presented to the endocrine clinic with weight gain, easy bruisability, and fatigue during the 3rd trimester of her pregnancy. On examination, she had high blood pressure and stria on the lower abdomen. Further blood investigations showed impaired glucose tolerance on oral glucose tolerance test. A clinical suspicion of Cushing's syndrome was raised and she underwent further evaluation.

    Which one of the following physiological changes is seen in ACTH-cortisol axis during normal pregnancy?
    A. Blunting of cortisol response to dexamethasone suppression test
    B. Loss of diurnal rhythm of cortisol secretion
    C. Lowered cortisol-binding globulin levels
    D. Lowered cortisol levels
    E. Urinary free cortisol levels five times the normal (non-pregnancy range)

11. **Glycoprotein hormones are characterized by a common α subunit and hormone-specific β subunit. In contrast, peptide hormones are synthesized from amino acids and typically generated as prohormones, which may be secreted in the circulatory system following a specific stimulus.**

    Which one of the following is a peptide hormone secreted in the human body under normal physiological state?

    A. Adrenocorticotropic hormone (ACTH)
    B. Follicle-stimulating hormone (FSH)
    C. Human chorionic gonadotropin (hCG)
    D. Luteinizing hormone (LH)
    E. Thyrotropin-stimulating hormone (TSH)

12. **A 54-year-old man presented to endocrine clinic with gradually worsening low mood, malaise, and reduced exercise capacity. He was known to have dyslipidaemia and ischaemic heart disease (IHD). He was operated on previously for a non-functioning pituitary adenoma (NFPA) resulting in partial anterior hypopituitarism, and had been on thyroxine and hydrocortisone replacement therapy. On examination, he had a BMI of 35 kg/m² with evidence of central adiposity.**

    ```
    Investigations:
      9 a.m. cortisol  415 nmol/L
      IGF-1            8 nmol/L (16-118)
      FT4              15.4 pmol/L (11.5-22.7)
      TSH              0.03 mU/L (0.35-5.5)
    ```

    Which one of the following tests is most appropriate in his case to confirm the diagnosis of adult GH deficiency?

    A. Domeperidone test
    B. GH levels
    C. Growth hormone releasing hormone (GHRH)-arginine stimulation test
    D. Insulin-like growth factor- binding protein IGFBP measurement
    E. Insulin tolerance test

13. **A 43-year-old teacher was reviewed in the endocrine clinic for symptoms of low mood and lethargy. She had undergone trans-sphenoidal resection of a NFPA 5 years ago, and was on thyroxine and hydrocortisone replacement therapy. She was also on zonisamide therapy for focal seizures.**

```
Investigations:
   prolactin  270 mU/L  (45-375)
   IGF-1      8 nmol/L  (16-118)
   FT4        15.4 pmol/L (11.5-22.7)
   TSH        0.03 mU/L (0.35-5.5)
```

Which one of the following tests is most appropriate to assess her suspected GH deficiency?

A. GH levels
B. Glucagon stimulation test
C. Glucose tolerance test
D. IGFBP3 levels
E. Insulin tolerance test

14. **A 66-year-old retired police officer presented to the endocrine clinic with low mood, reduced exercise tolerance, and malaise. He had undergone trans-sphenoidal resection of a NFPA 5 years ago and post-operatively developed partial anterior pituitary hormone deficiency. He also has a past medical history of prostate cancer (T2N0M0), which was cured by post-elective resection. At the time of presentation, he was on hydrocortisone, thyroxine, and testosterone replacement therapy.**

```
Investigations:
   IGF-1      6 nmol/L  (16-118)
   prolactin  186 mU/L  (45-375)
   FT4        16.5 pmol/L (11.5-22.7)
   TSH        0.11 mU/L (0.35-5.5)
   LFT        normal
```

Which one of the following is the most appropriate next step in his management?

A. Confirm the GH deficiency with a dynamic test
B. GH contra-indicated due to potential risk of tumour growth
C. Reduce thyroxine dose
D. Start GH therapy
E. Start octreotide

15. **A 52-year-old man presented to endocrine clinic with symptoms of reduced sexual drive. He smoked 5–6 cigarettes a day and denied use of any substance of abuse. On examination, he had a BMI of 45 kg/m² with evidence of central obesity and normal secondary sexual characteristic development with no anosmia.**

```
Investigations:
   FSH           1.5 U/L (1.4-18.1)
   LH            3.1 U/L (3-8)
   testosterone  5.5 nmol/L (8.5-28.5)
   MRI brain     normal pituitary gland
```

Which one of the following is the most likely aetiology for his reduced libido and hypogonadism?

A. Idiopathic

B. Increased BMI

C. Kallmann syndrome

D. Klinefelter's syndrome

E. Sheehan's syndrome

16. **A 65-year-old man presented to the accident and emergency unit with sudden-onset headache, nausea, and vomiting. On examination, he was drowsy with features of 3rd, 4th, and 6th cranial nerve palsy.**

    An urgent magnetic MRI brain was arranged (see Figure 1.1).

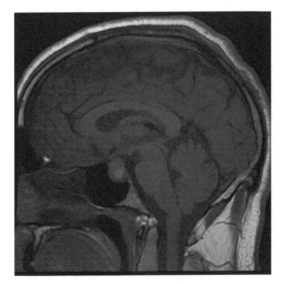

Figure 1.1 MRI pituitary gland sagittal view

All of the following are indications for urgent neurosurgical intervention in a patient with pituitary apoplexy except?

A. Deteriorating level of consciousness
B. Ocular paresis (3rd, 4th, and 6th cranial nerves)
C. Severe and persistent visual field defect
D. Severely reduced visual acuity
E. Worsening visual field defect

17. **A 17-year-old boy presented to the endocrine clinic with features of delayed puberty. On examination, he had a reduced sense of smell, small-sized testes, and under-developed secondary sexual characteristics.**

    ```
    Investigations:
      FSH            1.2 U/L (1.4-18.1)
      LH             1.5 U/L (3-8)
      testosterone   4.4 nmol/L (8.5-28.5)
      MRI brain      normal pituitary gland
    ```

    Which one of the following agents is the most useful therapeutic intervention to restore fertility in his clinical scenario?

    A. Cabergoline
    B. Clomiphene
    C. Gonadotropin-releasing hormones
    D. Octreotide
    E. Testosterone replacement

18. **A 26-year-old man was referred to the endocrine clinic with a history of decreased libido and erectile dysfunction. He confessed of having used an anabolic steroid 2 years previously for bodybuilding purposes. On examination, he was 1.85 m tall with a BMI of 25 kg/m². He had sparse facial and pubic hair, gynaecomastia, small testicles (right 2 mL and left 3 mL), and there was no anosmia.**

    ```
    Investigations:
      FSH            31 U/L (1.4-18.1)
      LH             12 U/L (3.0-8.0)
      testosterone   4.8 nmol/L (8.4-28.7)
      FT4            21.6 pmol/L (11.5-22.7)
      TSH            0.5 mu/L (0.35-5.5)
      prolactin      640 mU/L (100-550)
    ```

    Which one of the following is the most likely diagnosis in his clinical scenario?

    A. FSH-secreting pituitary adenoma (FSHoma)
    B. Kallmann syndrome
    C. Klinefelter's syndrome
    D. Prolactinoma
    E. Thyrotoxicosis

19. **An 18-year-old boy with idiopathic GH deficiency was reviewed in the adult endocrinology clinic for the first time. He had initially presented to the paediatric endocrinology clinic with delayed growth and was noticed to have features consistent with GH deficiency, which was subsequently confirmed with dynamic testing. He showed good response with GH replacement therapy.**

    ```
    Investigations:
      IGF-1       32 nmol/L (16-118)
      prolactin  225 mU/L (45-375)
      FT4         14.5 pmol/L (11.5-22.7)
      TSH         2.5 mU/L (0.35-5.5)
    ```

    Which one of the following is the most appropriate management approach when he is reviewed in adult endocrine clinic?

    A. Decrease the GH replacement dose
    B. Increase the GH replacement dose
    C. No change in GH replacement dose
    D. Stop the GH replacement
    E. Stop the GH replacement and reassess the GH axis

20. **A 48-year-old man presented to the endocrine clinic with symptoms of low mood, malaise, and loss of muscle mass. He was known to have partial anterior pituitary hormone deficiency and was on hydrocortisone, testosterone, and thyroxine replacement therapy.**

    ```
    Investigations:
      IGF-1        6 nmol/L (16-118)
      testosterone 14.5 nmol/L (9-25)
      FT4          18.4 pmol/L (11.5-22.7)
      TSH          0.04 mU/L (0.35-5.5)
    ```

    Which one of the following is the most appropriate step in his further management?

    A. Arrange arginine-GHRH stimulation test
    B. Arrange insulin tolerance test
    C. Increase thyroxine dose
    D. Reduce thyroxine dose
    E. Start GH replacement

21. **A 45-year-old woman with background history of growth hormone deficiency (GHD) is reviewed in the endocrine clinic on a routine visit. She had been on GH replacement therapy for the previous 1 year and had shown improvement in her quality of life as assessed by adult GHD assessment (AGHDA) scores.**

    Which one of the following metabolic changes is associated with GH replacement therapy?

    A. Decrease in exercise capacity

    B. Decrease in triglyceride levels

    C. Increase in bone mineral density

    D. Increase in low-density lipoprotein (LDL) cholesterol

    E. Unchanged lean body mass

22. **A 41-year-old woman presented to the accident and emergency department with a history of sudden-onset severe headache, nausea, vomiting, and visual disturbance. On examination, she was apyrexial, hypotensive, tachycardic with no features of meningism. She also had evidence of 3rd, 4th, and 6th cranial nerve palsies.**

MRI was arranged (see Figure 1.2).

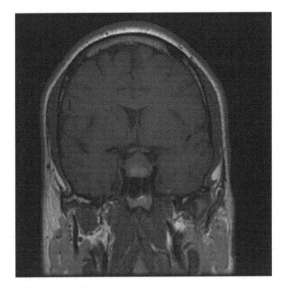

Figure 1.2 MRI pituitary gland coronal view

Which one of the following is a correct statement regarding the management of pituitary apoplexy?

A. Daily formal assessment of visual field and acuity is indicated in patients with reduced visual acuity or defective visual fields

B. Steroid therapy is indicated in patients, based on short synacthen test results

C. Surgical management is indicated in all patients, irrespective of severity of visual field defects.

D. Urgent neurosurgical intervention is indicated in all patients, with or without a significant decline in level of consciousness

E. Urgent neurosurgical intervention is indicated in patients with pituitary apoplexy showing ocular paresis.

23. **A 46-year-old nurse presented with symptoms of menstrual irregularities, lethargy, and mood swings. She had also noticed milky discharge from the nipples for the last 2 months. She was a known hypertensive, currently on amlodipine and doxazosin therapy. On examination, her visual fields were normal on confrontation testing.**

```
Investigations:
  FSH                        32 U/L (follicular 0.5-5, mid-
                             cycle 8-33, luteal 2-8)
  LH                         76 U/L (follicular 3-12, mid-
                             cycle 20-80, luteal 3-16)
  oestradiol                 18 pmol/L (follicular 17-260,
                             luteal 180-1100)
  IGF-1                      34 nmol/L (16-118)
  prolactin                  902 mU/L (45-375)
  FT4                        8.2 pmol/L (11.5-22.7)
  TSH                        16.8 mU/L (0.35-5.5)
  Urine for pregnancy test   negative
```

Which one of the following is the most likely explanation for her hyper-prolactinaemia and galactorrhoea?

A. Amlodipine

B. Doxazosin

C. Hypothyroidism

D. Prolactinoma

E. Menopause

24. **A 20-year-old university student presented with a 3-year history of ongoing menstrual irregularities and intermittent headaches. On examination, she had a BMI of 27 kg/m², with normal general physical and systemic examination, except for excessive facial hair growth.**

```
Investigations:
   FSH              5 U/L (follicular 0.5-5, mid-cycle 8-33,
                    luteal 2-8)
   LH               10 U/L (follicular 3-12, mid-cycle 20-80,
                    luteal 3-16)
   oestradiol       25 pmol/L (follicular 17-260, luteal
                    180-1100)
   prolactin        704 mU/L (45-375 mU/L)
   FT4              12.8 pmol/L (11.5-22.7)
   TSH              5.5 mU/L (0.35-5.5)
   testosterone  2.4 nmol/L (<1.5)
```

Which one of the following is the most likely cause for her elevated prolactin levels?

A. Hypothyroidism

B. Non-functional pituitary adenoma

C. Polycystic ovarian disease

D. Pregnancy

E. Prolactinoma

25. **A 26-year-old woman presented with a 4-month history of secondary amenorrhoea, episodic throbbing headache, together with visual symptoms (wavy lines and circles in front of eyes). She had a past medical history of microprolactinoma, diagnosed 4 years ago whilst being investigated for infertility, and had been on cabergoline therapy.**

```
Investigations:
   prolactin  1404 mU/L (45-375 mU/L)
   FT4        16.5 pmol/L (11.5-22.7 pmol/L)
   TSH        0.6 mU/L (0.35-5.5 mU/L)
```

Which one of the following is the most appropriate next step in her further management?

A. Switch to bromocriptine

B. Switch to quinagolide

C. Urgent MRI of the pituitary

D. Urgent visual field assessment

E. Take urine for pregnancy test

26. **A 31-year-old staff nurse with macroprolactinoma presented in the accident and emergency department with sudden-onset of headache and visual disturbance while she was 8 months pregnant. She had previously been on cabergoline therapy, which was stopped when her pregnancy was confirmed after an informed discussion.**

    An urgent visual field assessment showed no visual field defect.

    MRI of the pituitary showed an increase in size of prolactinoma in proximity to optic chiasm.

    Which one of the following is the most appropriate immediate step in her management?

    A. Induction of delivery
    B. Restart cabergoline therapy
    C. Start bromocriptine therapy
    D. Urgent neurosurgical intervention
    E. Urgent radiotherapy

27. **A 22-year-old woman was referred to the endocrine clinic with incidentally detected elevated prolactin levels, while she was being investigated for excessive facial hair growth. She had no history of galactorrhoea and her menstrual cycles were regular.**

    Her general physical and systemic examination was unremarkable.

    ```
    Investigations:
      IGF-1              18 nmol/L (16-118)
      prolactin          905 mU/L (60-620)
      free T₄            14.5 pmol/L (11.5-22.7)
      TSH                5.5 mU/L (0.35-5.5)
      9 a.m. cortisol   410 nmol/L
    ```

    MRI of the pituitary was inconclusive with midline pituitary stalk and no obvious lesion identified.

    Which one of the following is the most likely explanation for her elevated prolactin levels?

    A. Hook effect
    B. Hypothyroidism
    C. Infiltrative hypothalamic lesion
    D. Macroprolactin
    E. Non-functioning pituitary microadenoma

28. **A 28-year-old woman presented to endocrine clinic with secondary amenorrhoea and galactorrhoea for the last 6 months. Her general physical and systemic examination was normal.**

```
Investigations:
  Prolactin                3250 mU/L (60-620)
  Free T4                  15.5 pmol/L (11.5-22.7)
  TSH                      2.5 mU/L (0.35-5.5)
  Urine pregnancy test  Negative
```

MRI of the pituitary gland confirmed the presence of a microadenoma.

She was quite keen to start a family in the near future and sought advice regarding further management.

Which one of the following is the most appropriate therapeutic option in her case?

A. Bromocriptine
B. Elective trans-sphenoidal surgery
C. Octreotide
D. Quinagolide
E. Radiotherapy

29. **A 65-year-old woman presented to the diabetes clinic with worsening glycaemic control. She had recently been diagnosed with carpel tunnel syndrome and was awaiting an elective procedure. On examination, she had a coarse facial appearance, increased inter-dentate space, together with relatively big hands and feet.**

```
Investigations:
  IGF-1      102 nmol/L (16-118)
  prolactin  610 mU/L (45-375)
  FT4        12.5 pmol/L (11.5-22.7)
  TSH        1.5 mU/L (0.35-4.5)
```

Which one of the following is the most appropriate next step in her immediate management, while she is awaiting MRI of the pituitary gland?

A. Domperidone test
B. Glucose tolerance test
C. Insulin tolerance test
D. Start bromocriptine
E. Start cabergoline

30. **A 22-year-old woman known to have an aggressive GH tumour was reviewed in the endocrine clinic for further management. She was awaiting radiotherapy after incomplete cure achieved with trans-sphenoidal surgery. She had a strong family history of GH-secreting tumours.**

    Which one of the following mutations is associated with an increased risk of aggressive familial non-functioning and GH secreting pituitary adenomas?

    A. Aryl hydrocarbon receptor-interacting protein
    B. Menin
    C. *RET* proto-oncogene
    D. Succinate dehydrogenase B and D
    E. Succinate dehydrogenase C

31. **A 42-year-old college lecturer was reviewed in the endocrine clinic following trans-sphenoidal surgery for acromegaly, which was done about 8 months ago. Post-surgically there was an improvement in his symptoms, although the IGF-1 levels remained high and his glucose tolerance test showed unsuppressed GH levels suggestive of residual disease.**

    He was started on somatostatin analogue therapy, while awaiting repeat surgery.

    All of the following statements regarding development/management of colorectal polyps in patients with acromegaly are true except?

    A. An increased risk of colorectal adenomas
    B. An increased risk of colorectal cancer
    C. Repeat colonoscopy offered in patients with no polyp/normal IGF-1 every 10 years
    D. Repeat colonoscopy offered to patients with polyp and/or raised IGF-1 every 5 years
    E. Routine initial colonoscopy screening should begin at age of 50 years

32. A 45-year-old bus driver underwent elective trans-sphenoidal surgery for his GH-secreting macroadenoma. Post-operatively his IGF-1 levels remained elevated along with unsuppressed GH levels after the glucose tolerance test suggestive of an incomplete cure surgically.

He was started on somatostatin analogue therapy, but failed to respond. In view of the ongoing symptoms and raised IGF-1 levels he was considered for pegvisomant therapy while awaiting a multi-disciplinary team decision regarding repeat surgery or cranial irradiation.

Which one of the clinical/biochemical changes is associated with pegvisomant therapy?

A. Increase in GH levels
B. Increase in IGF-I levels
C. Increased risk of development of gall stones
D. Increased risk of pituitary tumour re-growth
E. Worsening of glycaemic control

33. A 17-year-old boy was referred to the endocrine clinic with features of short height and weight gain. On examination, he had increased BMI and central adiposity together with purple striae on lower abdomen.

```
Investigations:
  24 urine free cortisol/24 hours  268 nmol/24 hours (<146)
  11 p.m. salivary cortisol           6.5 nmol/L (<3.1)
  Low dose dexamethasone suppression test (LDDST)
  48-hour cortisol  380 nmol/L (<50)
  ACTH             56.7 ng/L (<51)
```

Which one of the following is the most appropriate next step in his management?

A. Bilateral inferior petrosal sinus sampling (BIPSS)
B. CT abdomen
C. CT abdomen and thorax
D. MRI of the pituitary
E. Octreotide scan

34. **A 52-year-old shop assistant presented with a 6-month history of diminishing exercise capacity and reduced libido. He was currently taking bisoprolol and terazosin tablets for blood pressure control.**

    His general physical and systemic examination was normal.

    ```
    Investigations:
        FSH             2.5 U/L  (1.4-18.1)
        LH              1.9 U/L  (3.0-8.0)
        testosterone    7.5 nmol/L (9-25)
        prolactin       855 mU/L (45-375)
        IGF-1           35 nmol/L (16-118)
        FT4             9.5 pmol/L (11.5-22.7)
        TSH             0.15 mU/L (0.35-5.5 mU/L)
    ```

    Which one of the following is the most likely cause for his elevated prolactin levels?

    A. Pituitary stalk compression
    B. Prolactinoma
    C. Secondary hypothyroidism
    D. Terazosin
    E. Thyrotoxicosis

35. **A 45-year-old lorry driver was referred to the endocrine clinic with symptoms of reduced libido and lack of energy. He had history of a traumatic head injury 5 years previously, which needed a period of 24 hours observation in hospital. On examination, his BMI was 42 kg/m^2, with normal general physical and systemic examination.**

    ```
    Investigations:
        free T₄         8.1 pmol/L (11.5-22.7)
        TSH             0.4 mU/L (0.35-5.5)
        FSH             2.2 U/L  (1.4-18.1)
        LH              3.5 U/L  (3.0-8.0)
        testosterone    6.8 nmol/L (8.4-28.7)
        IGF-1           35 nmol/L (16-118)
        prolactin       880 mU/L (45-375)
    ```

    Which one of the following is the most likely diagnosis, based on his clinical profile?

    A. Microprolactinoma
    B. Morbid obesity
    C. Non-functioning pituitary adenoma
    D. Post-traumatic pituitary apoplexy
    E. Primary hypothyroidism

36. The pituitary gland is composed of acidophilic (somatotrophs and lactotrophs) and basophilic (corticotrophs, thyrotrophs, gonadotrophs) or chromophobe cells based on histochemical staining with pH-dependent dyes.

    Which one of the following is generally the correct order of involvement of cells secondary to a compressive NFPA?

    A. Corticotrophs > thyrotrophs > somatotrophs > gonadotrophs
    B. Gonadotrophs > thyrotrophs > corticotrophs > somatotrophs
    C. Gonadotrophs > thyrotrophs > somatotrophs > corticotrophs
    D. Somatotrophs > gonadotrophs > thyrotrophs > corticotrophs
    E. Thyrotrophs > somatotrophs > corticotrophs > gonadotrophs

37. A 55-year-old woman presented to the clinic with symptoms of recurrent headaches and galactorrhoea. Her general physical and systemic examination was unremarkable. Her formal visual field assessment did not reveal any field defect. Her anterior pituitary hormone profile reassuringly showed results that are within normal range except from slightly elevated prolactin level.

    MRI of the pituitary gland confirmed the presence of a pituitary macroadenoma with extensive involvement of cavernous sinus.

    Which one of the following is the most appropriate management approach in her case?

    A. Cabergoline
    B. Conservative management
    C. Gamma knife radiosurgery
    D. Octreotide therapy
    E. Transfrontal craniotomy

38. **A 75-year-old retired army man was referred to the endocrine clinic with symptoms including recurrent headaches, lethargy, and malaise.**

His general physical and systemic examination was unremarkable.

```
Investigations:
    free T₄           6.8 pmol/L (11.5-22.7)
    TSH               0.5 mU/L (0.35-5.5)
    FSH               1.0 U/L (1.4-18.1)
    LH                2.5 U/L (3.0-8.0)
    testosterone      8.5 nmol/L (8.4-28.7)
    prolactin         655 mU/L (45-375)
    9 a.m. cortisol   381 nmol/L
```

MRI of the pituitary was undertaken (see Figure 1.3).

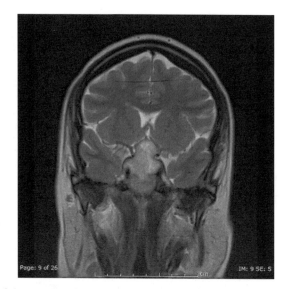

Figure 1.3 MRI of the pituitary gland—coronal view

Which one of the following is a definitive indication for elective surgery in a patient with NFPA?

A. Abnormal short synacthen test results

B. Optic chiasm compression

C. Recurrent headaches

D. Secondary hypothyroidism

E. Tumour size

39. **A 70-year-old man was referred to endocrine clinic with 6-week history of headache and visual disturbance. On examination, he had a bitemporal visual field defect, which was confirmed on formal visual field assessment.**

```
Investigations:
   free T₄         8.5 pmol/L (11.5-22.7)
   TSH             0.5 mU/L (0.35-5.5)
   FSH             1.0 U/L (1.4-18.1)
   LH              2.5 U/L (3.0-8.0)
   prolactin       800 mU/L (45-375)
   testosterone    3.5 nmol/L (8.4-28.7)
   9 a.m. cortisol 405 nmol/L
```

MRI showed a pituitary adenoma with suprasellar extension (see Figure 1.4).

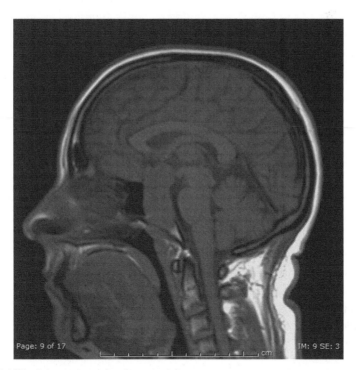

Figure 1.4 MRI of the pituitary gland—sagittal view

Which one of the following is the most appropriate definitive management approach for him?

A. Cabergoline therapy

B. Insulin tolerance test

C. Neurosurgical referral

D. Short synacthen test

E. Thyroxine and testosterone replacement

40. A 22-year-old woman presented with a history of menstrual irregularities for the previous 4 years. She had attained menarche at age of 13 years. Her general physical and systemic examination was unremarkable.

```
Investigations:
  FSH          45 U/L (follicular 0.5-5, mid-cycle 8-33,
               luteal 2-8)
  LH           2.5 U/L (follicular 3-12, mid-cycle 20-80,
               luteal 3-16)
  oestradiol   1332 pmol/L (follicular 17-260, luteal
               180-1100)
  prolactin    604 mU/L (45-375)
```

Ultrasound of pelvis showed bilateral enlarged and cystic ovaries. MRI of the pituitary showed an 18-mm pituitary tumour without any involvement of optic chiasm.

Which one of the following is the most likely diagnosis in her case?

A. Ectopic oestrogen-secreting tumour
B. Gonadotropin-secreting adenoma
C. Non-functioning pituitary adenoma
D. Ovarian hyper-stimulation syndrome
E. Polycystic ovarian syndrome with a pituitary incidentaloma

41. A 47-year-old post-menopausal woman presented to endocrine clinic with a 6-month history of palpitations, increasing shortness of breath, and weight loss. Her general physical and systemic examination was unremarkable.

Her thyroid function test (TFT) results were as shown:

```
FT4  24.8 pmol/L (9.0-19.1)
FT3  7.4 pmol/L (2.6-5.7)
TSH  6.15 mu/L (0.35-5.0)
```

Which one of the following clinical feature is inconsistent with a diagnosis of thyrotropinoma (TSHoma)?

A. α subunit/TSH ratio >1
B. Elevated sex hormone- binding globulin (SHBG) levels
C. Family history of thyroid problem
D. MRI pituitary showing macroadenoma.
E. Non-elevation of TSH after thyrotropin-releasing hormone (TRH) stimulation test

42. **A 66-year-old man presented with a 4-month history of weight loss, increased sweating, and palpitations. His general physical and systemic examination is unremarkable except for mild resting tremors. His TFT results are as shown:**

```
FT3  6.5 pmol/L (2.6-5.7)
FT4  25.0 pmol/L (11.5-22.7)
TSH  5.8 mU/L (0.35-5.5)
```

Which one of the following will be a useful test to establish the diagnosis?

A. α subunit to TSH ratio
B. Anti-TSH receptor antibodies
C. Octreotide scan
D. Thyroid ultrasound
E. Thyroid uptake scan

43. **An 85-year-old man was referred to the endocrine clinic with a 6-month history of weight loss, diarrhoea, and heat intolerance. He had a background history of IHD and severe congestive cardiac failure.**

His examination showed features of cachexia, bilateral tremors, and bi-basal crepitations on auscultation of lungs.

```
Investigations:
  free T4  26.5 pmol/L (11.5-22.7 pmol/L)
  free T3  9.1 pmol/L (3.5-6.5 pmol/L)
  TSH      8.5 mU/L (0.35-5.5 mU/L)
```

The remaining anterior pituitary hormone profile was within normal range. MRI of the pituitary showed a 15-mm pituitary adenoma, which was not compressing the optic chiasm. During the combined neurosurgical-endocrine multi-disciplinary team meeting, a decision was made to manage him with medical therapy, considering his co-morbidities.

Which one of the following is the treatment of choice for his further management?

A. Cabergoline
B. Carbimazole
C. Octreotide
D. Radioactive iodine (RAI) ablation
E. Radiotherapy

44. **Non-functioning pituitary adenoma are the commonest pituitary tumours, which account for approximately 90% of sellar masses, and may be detected incidentally or present with pressure symptoms.**

    Which one of the following is the commonest pattern/finding seen on immunostaining of a NFPA?

    A. Gonadotropins
    B. No immunostaining
    C. Non-specific immunostaining
    D. Prolactin
    E. Somatostatin

45. **A 36-year-old woman was incidentally detected to have a 6-mm pituitary micro-adenoma on a CT of the head arranged to evaluate cause for her recurrent headaches. Apart from the headaches that she had suffered for the last 6 months, she had no past history of any significant medical illness and was not on any regular medications. Her general physical and systemic examination was unremarkable.**

    Which one of the following is the most appropriate next step in her management?

    A. Anterior pituitary hormone profile
    B. Discharge from follow-up
    C. Formal visual field assessment
    D. Insulin tolerance test
    E. Neurosurgical referral

46. **A 41-year-old man was incidentally detected to have a pituitary tumour measuring 5 mm on a CT of the head done after a traumatic head injury. He had no significant past medical history and was not on any regular medications. His general physical and systemic examination was unremarkable.**

    ```
    Investigations:
      IGF-1              30 nmol/L (16-118)
      prolactin          262 mU/L (60-620)
      testosterone       9.4 nmol/L (8.5-28.5)
      free T₄            15.5 pmol/L (11.5-22.7)
      TSH                3.0 mU/L (0.35-5.5)
      9 a.m. cortisol    423 nmol/L
    ```

    Which one of the following is the most appropriate step with regard to his further management considering he remains asymptomatic?

    A. No follow-up required
    B. Repeat MRI of the pituitary after 4 months
    C. Repeat MRI of the pituitary after 1 year
    D. Repeat MRI of the pituitary/anterior pituitary hormone profile after 4 months
    E. Repeat MRI of the pituitary/anterior pituitary hormone profile after 1 year

47. **A 35-year-old woman was reviewed at the endocrine clinic on a follow-up visit. She was incidentally diagnosed as having a pituitary incidentaloma measuring 5 mm on investigations for a possible benign intracranial hypertension about 6 months ago. She complained of recurrent episodes of headache together with visual disturbance during this visit. On examination, she had bitemporal superior quadrantanopia.**

```
Investigations:
  IGF-1              12 nmol/L (16-118)
  prolactin          950 mU/L (60-620)
  free T₄            10.6 pmol/L (11.5-22.7)
  TSH                0.5 mU/L (0.35-5.5)
  9 a.m. cortisol    401 nmol/L
```

The repeat MRI scan showed significant increase in the size of pituitary tumour with compression of optic chiasm.

Which one of the following is the most appropriate next step in her management?

A. Cabergoline

B. Neurosurgical referral

C. Radiotherapy

D. Thyroxine

E. Thyroxine and GH therapy

48. **A 16-year-old was reviewed in a joint paediatrics to adult endocrinology transition clinic. He was diagnosed as having craniopharyngioma at age 14 years and underwent surgical removal of the tumour. Post-operatively, he was noticed to have delayed growth (as evidence by his height being 2 SDs below normal compared with other children his age). Both his parents were of average height and none of his siblings were of short stature.**

```
Investigations:
  0 hour cortisol            308 nmol/L
  30 minutes post-ACTH       592 nmol/L
  IGF-1                      12 nmol/L (16-118)
  prolactin                  145 mU/L (45-375)
  testosterone               11.2 nmol/L (8.5-28.5)
  TSH                        2.6 mU/L (0.35-5.5)
```

On insulin tolerance test a peak GH value of 9 mU/L (3 µg/L) was seen.

Which one of the following is the most appropriate approach for a potential GH therapy in his case?

A. Confirm the GH deficiency by a second dynamic test

B. GH replacement is contraindicated considering history of craniopharyngioma

C. Start on adult dose of GH replacement

D. Start on GH replacement only if he is symptomatic

E. Trial of GH therapy for 6 months only

49. **A 20-year-old woman was referred to the endocrine clinic with a history of persistent headache over the last 1 year. Her examination showed evidence of left temporal visual field defect. Subsequent anterior pituitary functions confirmed secondary hypothyroidism and hypogonadotrophic hypogonadism.**

    MRI of the pituitary showed a 4 × 2 cm cystic calcified para-sellar lesion, which was compressing the optic chiasm. The cysts were radiologically described as showing engine oil appearance.

    Which one of the following is the likely diagnosis based on her clinical profile?

    A. Craniopharyngioma
    B. Germinoma
    C. Neurosarcoidosis
    D. Pituitary adenoma
    E. Teratoma

50. **A 23-year-old woman presented to the endocrine clinic with a 6-week history of headaches, extreme fatigue, and malaise. She was in the post-partum period having delivered 3 months ago. Her general physical and systemic examination was unremarkable.**

    ```
    Investigations:
      0 hour cortisol                          55 nmol/L
      30-minute cortisol (post-synthetic 135 nmol/L
      ACTH injection)
      prolactin                                801 mu/L (100-550)
      FT4                                      9.2 pmol/L (11.5-22.7)
      TSH                                      0.1 mu/L (0.35-5.5)
    ```

    MRI of the pituitary showed an enhancing mass with thickening of the pituitary stalk and loss of posterior pituitary bright spot.

    Which one of the following is the most likely diagnosis?

    A. Histiocytosis
    B. Lymphocytic hypophysitis
    C. Neurosarcoidosis
    D. Pituitary adenoma
    E. Sheehan's syndrome

51. A 60-year-old man underwent elective trans-sphenoidal surgery for a non-functioning macroadenoma compressing optic chiasm. His post-operative recovery was uneventful.

Day 1, post-operative blood test results were as shown:

```
Na               144 mmol/L (135-145)
K                4.0 mmol/L (3.5-5.5)
urea             8.5 mg/dL (7-20)
creatinine       110 µmol/L (60-115)
free T₄          12.0 pmol/L (11.5-22.7)
TSH              0.8 mU/L (0.35-5.5)
9 a.m. cortisol  105 nmol/L
```

Which one of the following is the most appropriate immediate step in his management?

A. Formal visual field assessment

B. Hydrocortisone and thyroxine replacement

C. Hydrocortisone replacement

D. Insulin tolerance test

E. Observation

52. A 70-year-old man underwent elective trans-sphenoidal surgery for a NFPA, which was compressing the optic chiasm.

On post-operative day 3, he complained of polydipsia and polyuria. His urine output was noticed to be more than 5 L over a period of 24 hours.

```
Investigations:
  Na               148 mmol/L (135-145)
  K                4.6 mmol/L (3.5-5.5)
  urea             20.5 mg/dL (7-20)
  creatinine       124 µmol/L (60-115)
  calcium          2.71 mmol/L (2.2-2.6)
  random glucose   8.4 mmol/L
```

Which one of the following is the most likely aetiology for his symptoms?

A. Nephrogenic diabetes insipidus

B. Neurosarcoidosis

C. Primary hyperparathyroidism

D. Psychogenic polydipsia

E. Transient cranial diabetes insipidus

53. **A 55-year-old man complained of an intermittent clear discharge from the nose on a routine follow-up visit to the endocrine clinic. He was a known patient with NFPA who had undergone an elective trans-sphenoidal surgery about 6 weeks ago. Post-operatively he had developed a cerebrospinal fluid leak that required a surgical repair.**

    Which one of the following is the most appropriate step in his immediate management?

    A. Analyse the nasal discharge for β-transferrin
    B. CT angiogram
    C. ENT referral for nasal endoscopy
    D. MRI of the pituitary
    E. Urgent neurosurgical intervention

54. **A 45-year-old man was diagnosed as having acromegaly and underwent elective trans-sphenoidal surgery. Post-operatively his symptoms of headaches, sweating, and arthralgia persisted. His repeat IGF-1 levels remained elevated together with unsuppressed growth hormone levels on a glucose tolerance test. As a result, he was started on medical therapy in form of octreotide long-acting preparation injections and a repeat surgery was planned.**

    Which one of the following is a side effect/complication associated with octreotide treatment?

    A. Development of renal stones
    B. Impaired glycaemic control
    C. Increase in gall bladder contractility
    D. Increase in pituitary tumour size
    E. Increase in prolactin levels

55. **Pasireotide (SOM 230) is a somatostatin analogue, which is approved for treatment of adult patients with surgically incurable Cushing's disease. It has also been shown to be an efficacious agent in the medical management of patients with acromegaly.**

    Which one of the following clinical/physiological feature is associated with pasireotide (SOM 230) therapy?

    A. Increased risk of development of renal stones
    B. Increase in GH levels
    C. Increase in IGF-1
    D. Selective inhibition of somatostatin receptor subtype 2 and 4.
    E. Worsening of glycaemic control in patients with diabetes

56. **A 22-year-old university student presented to the endocrine clinic with 1-year history of secondary amenorrhoea. She also had symptoms of polydipsia and polyuria for the last 4 months.**

Her general physical and systemic examination was unremarkable.

Investigations:
```
  FSH                 6.0 U/L (follicular 0.5-5, mid-cycle 8-33,
                      luteal 2-8)
  LH                  3.3 U/L (follicular 3-12, mid-cycle 20-80,
                      luteal 3-16)
  Oestradiol          22 pmol/L (follicular 17-260, luteal
                      180-1100)
  Prolactin           775 mU/L (60-620)
  Free T₄             10.2 pmol/L (11.5-22.7 pmol/L)
  TSH                 0.5 mU/L (0.35-5.5 mU/L)
  9 a.m. Cortisol     352 nmol/L
Water deprivation test:
  Serum osmolality 298 mOsmol/Kg
  Urine osmolality 202 mOsmol/Kg at 6 hours
  Urine osmolality 780 mOsmol/Kg after desmopressin acetate
  (DDAVP)
```

Which one of the following is the likely diagnosis, based on the water deprivation test results?

A. Cranial diabetes insipidus

B. Nephrogenic diabetes insipidus

C. Normal results

D. Psychogenic polydipsia

E. Syndrome of inappropriate antidiuretic hormone secretion (SIADH)

57. **A 16-year-old boy presented to the endocrine clinic with symptoms of polydipsia and polyuria for the previous 6 months. He was known to have Type 1 diabetes (diagnosed at age 5 years) and developed severe visual impairment at age 10 years.**

His initial blood tests showed normal FBC, renal function, bone profile, and anterior pituitary function tests. His glycaemic control was good as reflected by a HbA1c of 50 mmol/mol.

```
Water deprivation test (at 6 hours):
  serum osmolality  300 mOsmol/Kg
  urine osmolality  220 mOsmol/Kg
  urine osmolality  830 mOsmol/Kg after DDAVP injection
```

Which one of the following is the likely inheritance pattern of his underlying condition?

A. Autosomal dominant

B. Autosomal recessive

C. Mitochondrial disease

D. Sporadic de novo mutation

E. X-linked

58. An 18-year-old student presented to the endocrine clinic with a 10-month history of secondary amenorrhoea. She also had developed symptoms of polydipsia and polyuria over the last 4 months. Her general physical and systemic examination was unremarkable.

```
Investigations:
  FSH                    5.5 U/L (follicular 0.5-5, mid-cycle
                         8-33, luteal 2-8)
  LH                     2.8 U/L (follicular 3-12, mid-cycle
                         20-80, luteal 3-16)
  oestradiol             32 pmol/L (follicular 17-260, luteal
                         180-1100)
  prolactin              990 mU/L (60-620)
  9 a.m. cortisol        400 nmol/L
  fasting blood glucose  5.5 mmol/L
  serum calcium          2.35 mmol/L (2.2-2.6)
Water deprivation test:
  Serum osmolality  301 mOsmol/Kg
  Urine osmolality  205 mOsmol/Kg at 6 hours
  Urine osmolality  805 mOsmol/Kg after DDAVP
```

Her MRI pituitary showed a homogenous solid enhancing mass, involving the hypothalamus and pituitary stalk. There was no cystic area and a differential diagnosis of germinoma versus hypophysitis (lymphocytic/granulomatous) was considered.

Which one of the following investigations may be helpful to distinguish a germinoma from hypophysitis?

A. β-transferrine test

B. Serum/CSF β-hCG and α-foetoprotein levels

C. Domperidone test

D. Serum cerruloplasmin levels

E. Ultrasound pelvis/ovaries

59. **A 42-year-old woman was referred by her GP with symptoms of excessive tiredness, arthralgia, increased sweating, and weight gain. She had a background medical history of primary autoimmune hypothyroidism and was taking levothyroxine tablets.**

    She had noticed a change in her facial appearance (see Figures 1.5 and 1.6).

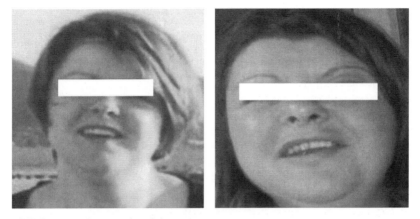

Figure 1.5 Previous photographs of the patient

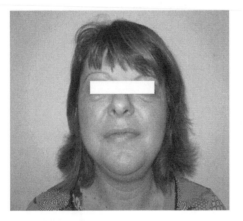

Figure 1.6 Latest photograph of the patient

Which one of the following is most appropriate next step to help establish the underlying diagnosis?

A. IGF-1 levels and oral glucose tolerance test
B. Insulin tolerance test
C. Low-dose dexamethasone test
D. Prolactin levels
E. Water deprivation test

60. **A 45-year-old woman presented to the endocrine clinic with a change in size of her ring, increased sweating, and change in facial appearance over the last 1 year. She was a known patient with type 2 diabetes mellitus and had noticed a worsening of glycaemic control. On examination, she had coarse facial features, prognathism, and macroglossia.**

```
Investigations:
    FSH           6.5 U/L (1.4-18.1)    IGF-1  170 nmol/L (16-118)
    LH            5.4 U/L (3.0-8.0)     FT4    12.6 pmol/L (11.5-22.7)
    testosterone  7.5 nmol/L (9-25)     TSH    3.6 mU/L (0.35-5.5 mU/L)
    prolactin     2800 mU/L (45-375)
```

Oral glucose tolerance test results:

Time (minutes)	Growth hormone	Plasma glucose
0	6.21	6.4
30	6.49	10.8
60	8.78	8.5
90	9.88	6.8
120	12	5.2

See Figure 1.7.

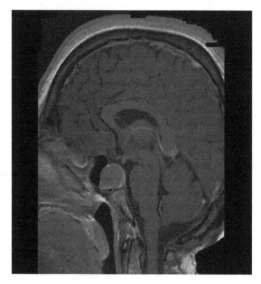

Figure 1.7 MRI of the pituitary—sagittal view

Reproduced with permission from Dr S. Rice, Consultant Endocrinologist, Hywel Dda University Health Board, Llanelli

Which one of the following is the most appropriate immediate step in her management?

A. Cabergoline
B. Hydrocortisone
C. Pegvisomant
D. Somatostatin analogues
E. Urgent trans-sphenoidal surgery

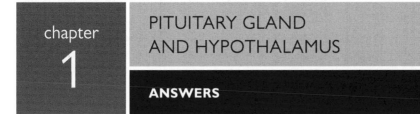

1. D. Somatotrophs constitute around 50% of anterior pituitary cell population (See Table 1.1). These are generally acidophilic.

Table 1.1 Various cell population of pituitary gland with their staining characteristics

Relative % of cell types in the pituitary	Acidophilic staining	Basophil staining	Hormones secreted
50%	Somatotrophs		GH
10–25%	Lactotrophs		Prolactin
15–20%		Corticotrophs	ACTH, POMC, endorphins, lipotrophin
10–15%		Gonadotrophs	FSH, LH
10%		Thyrotrophs	TSH

Melmed S. The pituitary (3rd edn). Academic Press/Elsevier, 2011.

2. D. The cotricotrophs are basophilic and PAS positive due to high glycoprotein content. They also secrete β endorphins. The gonadotrophs and thyrotrophs are also basophil staining. The lactotrophs and somatotrophs are acidophilic.

Gardner D & Shoback D. Greenspan's basic and clinical endocrinology (9th edn). Lange Publishers, 2011.

Melmed S. The pituitary (3rd edn). Academic Press/Elsevier, 2011.

3. C. Pro-opio-melano-corticotropin (POMC) serves as a precursor for the ACTH, β-endorphins, and melatonin release. ACTH secretion is increased by CRH, vasoactive intestinal peptide, catecholamines, and ghrelin, while oxytocin, endocannabinoids, and atrial natriuretic peptide decrease its secretion.

Hill M, Patel S, Campolongo P, et al. Functional Interactions between stress and the endocannabinoid system: from synaptic signaling to behavioral output. Journal of Neuroscience, 2010; 30(45):14980–14986.

Hill M & Tasker J. Endocannabinoid signaling, glucocorticoid-mediated negative feedback and regulation of the HPA axis. Neuroscience. 2012; 204: 5–16.

4. E. The highest level of GH secretion is seen in sleep, in contrast to the lowest level of cortisol attained around midnight. The level of GH secretion decreases by around 10–15% with every decade of life. Exercise and a loss of weight are associated with an increase in GH levels. Hypoglycaemia is an extremely potent stimulus for GH secretion.

The GH levels increase in malnutrition in contrast to a decrease in IGF-1 levels. High blood glucose is associated with an initial suppression (for 1–3 hours) of GH levels (postulated to be due to somatostatin-mediated inhibition of GH secretion) followed by a rise (postulated to be due to a reciprocal increase in GHRH release and decrease in somatostatinergic tone).

An increase in GH levels is seen in patients with Type 1 diabetes mellitus (DM), while in patients with Type 2 DM the levels may be increased, normal or decreased. This is probably a reflection of the contrasting influence of increased BMI and high blood glucose values on GH levels in this cohort of patients.

Gardner D & Shoback D. Greenspan's basic and clinical endocrinology (9th edn). Lange Publishers, 2011.

5. C. Ghrelin stimulates secretion of GH, insulin, ACTH, and prolactin. It has orexigenic properties (promotes feeding) and enhances gastric emptying. It also modulates the use of metabolic substrates, with ghrelin null mice displaying an increase utilization of fat as a substrate.

Dezaki K. Ghrelin function in insulin release and glucose metabolism. Endocrine Development 2013; 25: 135–143.

Inui A, Asakawa A, Bowers C, et al. Ghrelin, appetite, and gastric motility: the emerging role of the stomach as an endocrine organ. FASEB Journal, 2004; 18(3): 439–456.

Murray C, Martin N, Patterson M, et al. Ghrelin enhances gastric emptying in diabetic gastroparesis: a double blind, placebo controlled, crossover study. Gut, 2005; 54: 1693–1698.

6. C. Vasopressin mediates its physiological effects by acting on vasopressin receptors. There are three major types of vasopressin receptors:

- V1a: mediates smooth muscle contraction, platelet adhesion and increased glycogenolysis; present on vascular smooth muscles, platelets and liver.
- V1b: mediates ACTH release; present on corticotrophs (anterior pituitary gland).
- V2: mediates increased aquaporin 2 synthesis and assembly, leading to reabsorption of water from distal nephron.

Gardner D and Shoback D. Greenspan's basic and clinical endocrinology (9th edn). Lange Publishers, 2011.

Sharman A and Low J. Vasopressin and its role in critical care. Continuing Education in Anaesthesia Critical Care & Pain, 2008; 8(4): 134–137.

7. A. Advancing age is associated with an increased vasopressin release, together with decreased thirst perception and reduced fluid intake. An increased vasopressin secretion is seen in hypovolaemia, blood loss, and hypotension mediated via vasopressin V1a receptors. A decrease in ADH secretion may be seen with genetic conditions (Wolfram syndrome), tumours (Craniopharyngioma, Germinoma), and inflammatory conditions (Sarcoidosis, Histiocytosis).

Gardner D and Shoback D. Greenspan's basic and clinical endocrinology (9th edn). Lange Publishers, 2011.

Sharman A and Low J. Vasopressin and its role in critical care. Continuing Education in Anaesthesia Critical Care & Pain, 2008; 8(4): 134–137.

8. A. Oxytocin has been postulated to have varied physiological functions, such as its role in increasing uterine contractions, facilitation of child birth (cervical and uterine dilatation), social recognition, mating, and maternal bonding. It is not deemed necessary for lactation in women, as is seen in women lacking the posterior pituitary who can have normal lactation despite the absence of oxytocin secretion.

Gimpl G and Fahrenholz F. The oxytocin receptor system: structure, function and regulation. Physiological reviews, 2001; 81(2): 629–683.

9. C. Pasireotide, a newer somatostatin analogue has the highest affinity for SSTR-2 and SSTR-5, which are the most prevalent SSTR expressed on GH-secreting pituitary adenomas.

Lesche S, Lehmann D, Nagel F, et al. Differential effects of octreotide and pasireotide on somatostatin receptor internalization and trafficking in vitro. Journal of Clinical Endocrinology and Metabolism, 2009; 94(2): 654–661.

10. A. Normal physiological changes in pregnancy include weight gain; development of stria; an increase in levels of cortisol-binding globulin levels, resulting in increased cortisol levels; increased urinary free cortisol levels (up to 3-fold compared with the non-pregnant state during late third trimester) together with failure of dexamethasone to suppress cortisol response. There is no change in the circadian rhythm of cortisol secretion. Low or high dose dexamethasone suppression test and/or CRH stimulation may be employed to distinguish physiological changes associated with pregnancy from Cushing's syndrome. Reassuringly, Cushing's syndrome is extremely uncommon in pregnancy.

Jung C, Torpy D, Rogers A, et al. A longitudinal study of plasma and urinary cortisol in pregnancy and postpartum. Journal of Clinical Endocrinology and Metabolism, 2011; 96(5): 1533–1540.

Lim W, Torpy D, and Jeffries W. The medical management of Cushing's syndrome during pregnancy. European Journal of Obstetrics & Gynecology and Reproductive Biology, 2012; 1(168): 1–6.

11. A. ACTH is a single chain polypeptide cleaved from pro-opio-melanocortin. The rest of the hormones mentioned are examples of glycoprotein hormones, which share a common α subunit.

Melmed S. The pituitary (3rd edn). Academic press Elsevier, 2011.

12. C. Growth hormone is secreted in a pulsatile manner with around 5 pulses of hormone secretion in a period of 24 hours. The highest level of GH secretion is seen around midnight during the sleep period. A random measurement of GH secretion is not useful due to the pulsatile nature of secretion. The clinical features of growth hormone deficiency (GHD) are non-specific and include lethargy, low mood, poor quality of life, loss of muscle mass, and central adiposity. A low IGF-1 in such a clinical context may point towards GHD, which needs to be confirmed with dynamic tests for GH secretion.

Insulin tolerance test (ITT) is considered the gold standard for assessing GH secretion, although it needs to be conducted carefully in a closely-monitored space due to the risks associated with hypoglycaemia. ITT is contra-indicated in patients with seizures or IHD. As a result, an alternative test such as arginine-GHRH stimulation test is employed (as in this clinical scenario where the patient has IHD). About 30–40% of patients with GHD may have a normal IGF-1 level. IGF-1 levels are influenced by age, time of onset of GHD, and degree of hypopituitarism. The dynamic tests for GH assessment are not influenced with advancing age, although there is a 10–15% decline in GH secretion with every decade of life. Increased BMI blunts the GH response to insulin and obese patients are vulnerable to have a false positive test with insulin tolerance test. A peak GH response of <9 mU/L (<3 ng/mL) is suggestive of severe GHD.

Molitch ME, Clemmons DR, Malozowski S, et al. Evaluation and treatment of adult growth hormone deficiency: an endocrine society clinical practice guidelines. Journal of Clinical Endocrinology and Metabolism, 2011; 96(6): 1587–1609.

13. B. The gold standard for diagnosis of GH secretion is the ITT. GH levels of <3 µg/L (<10 mU/L) are usually indicative of severe GH deficiency on ITT. The contraindications for ITT include history of epilepsy IHD and basal cortisol levels <100 nmol/L. ITT is contraindicated in this patient as she has epilepsy and taking zonisamide therapy. Glucagon stimulation test can also be used for GH deficiency assessment if ITT is contraindicated (see Table 1.2).

Table 1.2 The sensitivity and specificity of various dynamic tests used for diagnosis of GH deficiency

Test	Sensitivity	Specificity
ITT	96%	92%
GHRH-arginine test	95%	91%
IGF-1	70%	80%
IGFBP3	50–70%	95%

Cook D, Yuen K, Miller B, et al. Guidelines for use of growth hormone in clinical practice (2009, update). Endocrine Practice, 2009; 15(Suppl. 2).

Molitch ME, Clemmons DR, Malozowski S, et al. Evaluation and treatment of adult growth hormone deficiency: an endocrine society clinical practice guidelines. Journal of Clinical Endocrinology and Metabolism, 96(6): 1587–1609.

14. D. This patient has features of GH deficiency as evidenced by his symptoms and low IGF-1 levels. A low IGF-1 level in the presence of 3 or more anterior pituitary hormone deficiencies (in an otherwise well-nourished healthy male with normal liver function) is a strong predictor of GH deficiency. A confirmatory dynamic test to assess GH reserve is not necessarily warranted in this scenario.

Presence of an active malignancy is a contra-indication to GH replacement therapy. There is no evidence of potential de novo tumour development or growth of pituitary/parasellar tumour growth with GH replacement therapy.

Glynn N and Agha A. Diagnosing growth hormone deficiency in adults. International Journal of Endocrinology, 2012 (2012): Article ID 976217.

15. B. Testosterone production is under control of LH, while sperm production is controlled by FSH. The release of both LH and FSH is regulated by pulsatile secretion of gonadotropin-releasing hormone (GnRH) secreted by hypothalamus. This gentleman has hypogonadotrophic hypogonadism as reflected by low testosterone and inappropriately low normal FSH and LH levels. A normal MRI rules out any structural lesion involving pituitary gland or hypothalamus. Increased BMI is associated with an increased aromatase activity in adipose tissues, which in turn leads to enhanced conversion of testosterone to oestradiol as a result gonadotropin secretion is suppressed through the negative feedback. See Table 1.3.

Table 1.3 Major causes of hypogonadotrophic hypogonadism

Aetiology	Example
Genetic disorders	Kallmann syndrome, transcription factor mutations, such as DAX1, Prop 1.
GnRH related	GnRH releasing hormone deficiency and/or GnRH receptor mutation.
Structural disorders	Pituitary-adenoma, craniopharyngioma, germinoma
Iatrogenic	Post-surgical or post-cranial irradiation
Organic	Excessive exercise, systemic illness, obesity, anorexia nervosa, stress, anabolic steroids, recreational drugs
Infiltrative disease	Sarcoidosis, haemochromatosis
Congenital syndromes	Laurence–Moon–Biedl, Prader–Willi syndrome
Hyperprolactinaemia or oestrogen excess	Prolactinoma, oestrogen-secreting tumour, oral contraceptive pills
Miscellaneous	HIV infection, chronic alcohol abuse, cirrhosis

Dandona P and Dhindsa S. Update: hypogonadotropic hypogonadism in type 2 diabetes and obesity. Journal of Clinical Endocrinology and Metabolism, 2011; 96(9): 2643–2651.

Silveira L and Latronico A. Approach to patients with hypogonadotropic hypogonadism. Journal of Clinical Endocrinology & Metabolism 2013; 98(5), 1781–1788.

16. B. Pituitary apoplexy is a medical emergency characterized by sudden onset of headache, nausea, and vomiting, with or without reduced visual acuity/visual field defect (bitemporal hemianopia) and ocular palsies (2nd, 3rd, 4th, and 6th nerves) secondary to a haemorrhage and/or an infarction in pituitary gland. A detailed history should focus on pre-existing pituitary dysfunction. Anterior pituitary function including FT4, TSH, IGF-1, random cortisol, prolactin, gonadotropins, and oestrogen (in women) and testosterone (in men) should be checked on an urgent basis. Patients who are haemodynamically unstable should be started on hydrocortisone therapy empirically. MRI of the pituitary is the radiological modality of choice to confirm the diagnosis.

The indications for urgent neurosurgical intervention include:

- Worsening of level of consciousness.
- Severely reduced visual acuity.
- Severe, persistent, and/or worsening visual field defects.

The presence of ocular palsy in the absence of visual field defect or reduced visual acuity is not an indication to urgent surgical intervention.

Rajasekaran S, Vanderpump M, Baldeweg S, et al. UK guidelines for the management of pituitary apoplexy. Pituitary Apoplexy Guidelines Development Group: May 2010. Clinical Endocrinology, 2011; 74: 9–20.

17. C. The presence of pubertal delay together with anosmia in this boy is suggestive of a diagnosis of Kallmann syndrome. Mutations in *KAL1*, *DAX1*, GnRH receptor, *PC1*, and *GPR54* (a gene encoding G protein coupled receptor binding kisseptin 1) have been linked to development of Kallmann syndrome and idiopathic hypogonadotrophic hypogonadism.

Patients with suspected Kallmann syndrome should have anterior pituitary hormone profile and MRI pituitary to rule out structural/anatomical pituitary/hypothalamic anomalies. Serum ferritin should be assessed in adult onset hypogonadotrophic hypogonadism to rule out haemochromatosis. Semen analysis should be arranged in male patients with Kallmann syndrome for assessment of potential fertility.

Testosterone replacement therapy is useful to improve libido, muscle mass, development of secondary sexual characteristics and prevent osteoporosis. Pulsatile GnRH therapy is helpful to restore hypothalamic-pituitary-gonadal function and fertility. Alternatively, patients can be started on gonadotropins (β-hCG) therapy to restore fertility.

Smith N and Quniton R. Kallmann syndrome: a patient's journey. British Medical Journal 2012; 345: e6971.

18. C. He has hypergonadotrophic hypogonadism (primary hypogonadism) with small testicles. Patients with Klinefelter syndrome may have mild elevation of prolactin levels. Phenotypically, they are tall and at puberty usually have compensated primary hypogonadism.

Blevins C and Wilson M. Klinefelter's syndrome. British Medical Journal, 2012; 345: e7558.

Radicioni A, Ferlin A, Balercia G, et al. Consensus statement on diagnosis and clinical management of Klinefelter syndrome. Journal of Endocrinology Investigations, 2010; 33(11): 839–850.

19. E. GHD in childhood may be an isolated defect or occur in the presence of other anterior pituitary hormonal defects. An isolated GHD in turn may be due to structural pituitary defects (e.g. craniopharyngioma), genetic mutations, and post-cranial irradiation therapy or due to partial deficiency of GHRH.

The children with isolated GHD and structurally normal pituitary can potentially recover spontaneously. As a result, children with idiopathic GH deficiency should have their GH replacement therapy stopped at the end of linear growth and re-assessment of GH secretion using dynamic tests.

Maghnie M, Stigazzi C, Tinelli C, et al. Growth hormone (GH) deficiency of childhood onset: Reassessment of GH status and evaluation of the predictive criteria for permanent GH deficiency in young adults. Journal of Endocrinology and Metabolism, 1999; 84(4): 1324–1328.

Stanley T. Diagnosis of growth hormone deficiency in childhood. Current Opinion in Endocrinology and Diabetes Obesity, 2012; 19(1): 47–52.

20. E. In the presence of three or more anterior pituitary hormonal defects, GH replacement therapy can be started without the need to arrange dynamic tests for the GH axis if the IGF-1 levels are low in the right clinical context. This patient has low TSH and a normal FT4 level, while being on thyroxine therapy. His low TSH is a reflection of pituitary structural/secretory defect (postoperative in this scenario). The thyroxine dose need to be titrated based on FT4 levels, rather than TSH values in secondary hypothyroidism.

NICE guidelines (TA 64) human GH (somatropin) replacement in adults with GH deficiency.

21. C. GH replacement therapy is associated with an increase in bone mineral density, reduction in total body fat and increase in lean body mass. It is associated with a decrease in LDL-cholesterol, increase in HDL-cholesterol with minimal or no impact on triglyceride concentrations. The side effects associated with GH replacement include headache, nausea, vomiting, arthralgia, and fluid retention. Rarely patients may develop benign intracranial hypertension and papilloedema. The dose of GH replacement therapy is titrated based on patient response and IGF-1 levels.

Vijaykumar A, Novosyadlyy R, Wu Y, et al. Biological effects of growth hormone on carbohydrate and lipid metabolism. Growth Hormone and IGF Research, 2010; 20(1): 1.

22. A. Daily formal assessment of visual field and acuity is indicated in patients with reduced visual acuity or defective visual fields. Empirical steroid therapy should be started in haemodynamically unstable patients with suspected pituitary apoplexy without awaiting the results of short synacthen test results. Surgical intervention is indicated in patients with severe or persistent visual field defects and/or in patients showing significant decline in level of consciousness. Ocular palsies due to 3rd, 4th, and 6th cranial nerve involvement is not an indication for surgery, as these are expected to recover over a course of time,

Rajasekaran S, Vanderpump M, Baldeweg S, et al. UK guidelines for the management of pituitary apoplexy. Pituitary Apoplexy Guidelines Development Group: May 2010. Clinical Endocrinology, 2011; 74: 9–20.

23. C. Severe hypothyroidism can potentially lead to hyper-prolactinaemia due to increased levels of thyrotropin-releasing hormone (TRH), which acts as a prolactin releasing factor. The treatment of underlying hypothyroidism with thyroxine therapy generally brings about improvement in prolactin levels.

24. C. The presence of menstrual irregularities along with elevated testosterone levels points towards a diagnosis of polycystic ovarian disease, which can be associated with mildly increased prolactin. She is also on oral contraceptive pills, which can lead to hyperprolactinaemia. Oestrogen directly stimulates lactotrophs leading to increased prolactin synthesis and secretion.

25.E. Women with a prolactinoma commonly present with menstrual irregularities (amenorrhoea, or oligomenorrhoea, or occasionally menorrhagia) together with infertility due to anovulatory cycles. The use of cabergoline is associated with the normalization of prolactin levels and gonadal function, which may result in the restoration of fertility. Patients who are started on ca-bergoline therapy and do not want pregnancy should be offered advice regarding contraception. A patient with secondary amenorrhoea while being on cabergoline therapy should stop taking the tab-lets and take a urine pregnancy test. Cabergoline therapy has not been associated with an increased number of abortions or congenital malformations, according to the current available evidence.

Colao A, Abs R, Barcena D, et al. Pregnancy outcomes following cabergoline treatment: extended results from a 12-year observational study. Clinical Endocrinology (Oxford), 2008; 68(1): 66–71.

Lebbe M, Hubinont C, Bernard P, et al. Outcome of 100 pregnancies initiated under treatment with cabergoline in hyperprolactinaemic women. Clinical Endocrinology (Oxford), 2010; 73(2): 236–242.

26. B. There is <5% and 15–40% probability of re-growth of a microprolactinoma and macro-prolactinoma, respectively, during pregnancy. The management of a macroprolactinoma during pregnancy is challenging as measurement of prolactin can be unreliable. The patients need to be monitored closely with periodic formal assessment of visual fields. In this patient, although the tumour is showing growth the visual fields are not affected as a result an urgent neurosurgical inter-vention is not indicated and cabergoline therapy can be restarted.

Cabergoline is not associated with any increase number of abortions or congenital malformations according to the current available evidence. An urgent trans-sphenoidal resection of tumour can be considered if the tumour fails to respond to cabergoline therapy and/or patient shows worsening of visual field related symptoms due to progressive chiasmal compression.

Colao A, Abs R, Barcena D, et al. Pregnancy outcomes following cabergoline treatment: extended results from a 12-year observational study. Clinical Endocrinology (Oxford), 2008; 68(1): 66–71.

Lebbe M, Hubinont C, Bernard P, et al. Outcome of 100 pregnancies initiated under treatment with cabergoline in hyperprolactinaemic women. Clinical Endocrinology (Oxford), 2010; 73(2): 236–242.

27. D. A normal menstrual cycle in the presence of mildly elevated prolactin with normal pituitary gland and the absence of symptoms makes it unlikely to be a prolactinoma. Macroprolactin with its longer half-life and biologically inert nature needs to be measured, although most laboratories auto-matically check for macroprolactin levels above certain levels or threshold.

Suliman A, Smith T, Gibney J, et al. Frequent misdiagnosis and mismanagement of hyperprolactinemic patients before the introduction of macroprolactin screening: application of a new strict laboratory definition of macroprolactinemia. Clinical Chemistry, 2003; 49(9): 1504–1509.

Vaishya R, Gupta R, and Arora S. Macroprolactin; a frequent cause of misdiagnosed hyperprolactine-mia in clinical practice. Journal of Reproductive Infertility, 2010; 11(3): 161–167.

28. A. Bromocriptine is a safe option for females in the reproductive age group presenting with a microprolactinoma if they are planning pregnancy in near future. The therapy can be stopped once the patient conceives and pregnancy is confirmed. The dopamine agonists help reduce prolactin levels and induce ovulation. Therefore, if pregnancy is not desired women should be given advice regarding contraception on the initiation of therapy. Cabergoline use in pregnant women has also not been associated with any increased risk of foetal malformation based on current available data.

Casanueva F, Molitch M, Schlechte J, et al. Guidelines of the Pituitary Society for the diagnosis and management of prolactinomas. Clinical Endocrinology (Oxford), 2006; 65(2): 265–267.

29. B. This patient has acromegalic features; a normal IGF-1 level does not exclude the diagnosis of acromegaly. OGTT with GH measurements remains the gold standard for the diagnosis of ac-romegaly with a failure to suppress GH level to <0.4 ng/mL supportive of the diagnosis. The GH secreting tumours are generally >10 mm in size and, as the clinical impact of excess GH secretion is often subtle, there may be a lag of 5–6 years before the diagnosis of acromegaly is confirmed. The elevated prolactin in this patient is more probably caused by stalk compression due to a GH secreting pituitary adenoma.

Katznelson L, Atkinson J, Cook D, et al. American association of clinical endocrinologists medical guidelines for clinical practice for the diagnosis and treatment of acromegaly—2011 update. Endocrine Practice, 2011; 17(Suppl. 4).

30. A. Aryl hydrocarbon receptor-interacting protein (AIP) mutation is associated with development of 15–20% of familial isolated pituitary adenomas (FIPA), an autosomal dominant disease with low penetrance. AIP mutation positive patients usually have invasive GH, mixed GH, and prolactin or prolactin-secreting macroadenoma. The tumours in patients with these mutations are generally more aggressive and present at a relatively younger age (mean age at diagnosis: 20–24 years).

Beckers A, Aaltonen L, Daly A, et al. Familial isolated pituitary adenomas (FIPA) and the pituitary adenoma predisposition due to mutations in the aryl hydrocarbon receptor interacting protein (AIP) gene. Endocrine Reviews, 2013; 34(2): 239–277.

31. E. The patients with acromegaly are at an increased risk of developing colorectal polyps and carcinoma. The polyps are often multiple, dysplastic, and more commonly found in the right side of the colon. The routine initial colonoscopy screening is recommended from the age of 40 years. In case there is no polyp and no active disease (based on clinical profile and normal IGF-1 values) a repeat colonoscopy should be offered to the patients at every 10-year interval. In patients with benign polyp (and/or raised IGF-1, active disease) on initial colonoscopy, it needs to be repeated every 5 years.

Jenkins P and Fairclough P. Screening guidelines for colorectal cancer and polyps in patients with acromegaly. Gut, 2002; 51: v13–v14.

Katznelson L, Atkinson J, Cook D, et al. American association of clinical endocrinologists medical guidelines for clinical practice for the diagnosis and treatment of acromegaly—2011 update. Endocrine Practice, 2011; 17(Suppl. 4).

32. A. Pegvisomant is a genetically-modified analogue of GH, which acts as a highly selective GH receptor, which is useful for patients who are resistant or intolerant to somatostatin analogue therapy. It has a higher affinity for GH receptors site 1. It is used as a subcutaneous injection and the higher cost of therapy is a major limitation for its widespread use. It leads to the normalization of IGF-1 levels in more than 90% of patients with no adverse impact on glycaemic control or glucose tolerance as compared with the somatostatin analogues. It leads to an increase in GH levels through a loss of negative feedback effect. It does not lead to any shrinkage in tumour size.

Madsen M, Fisker S, Feldt-Rasmussen U, et al. Circulating levels of pegvisomant and endogenous growth hormone during prolonged pegvisomant therapy in patients with acromegaly. Clinical Endocrinology (Oxford), 2014; 80(1): 92–100.

33. D. Cushing's syndrome can present in children and young adults with an increase in body weight, central obesity, and growth retardation. Adrenal tumours are relatively more common as a cause of ACTH-independent Cushing's syndrome in children younger than age 10 and may have associated signs of virilization. Cushing's disease due to a pituitary tumour (ACTH secreting) is more common in older children. Ectopic ACTH production due to a bronchogenic malignancy or neuroendocrine tumour is extremely rare in this age group. This patient had a measurable ACTH level in presence of hypercortisolism. His LDDST showed unsuppressed cortisol levels. An MRI pituitary is the next step in his management and BIPSS should only be considered if MRI pituitary results are equivocal.

Keil M and Stratakis C. Pituitary tumors in childhood: an update in their diagnosis, treatment and molecular genetics. Expert Review of Neurotherapeutics, 2008; 8(4): 563–574.

Nieman L, Biller B, Findling J, et al. The diagnosis of Cushing's syndrome: an endocrine society clinical practice guideline. Journal of Clinical Endocrinology & Metabolism, 2008; 93(5): 1526–1540.

34. A. The presence of an elevated prolactin level along with secondary hypothyroidism and hypogonadism is indicative of stalk compression due to pituitary adenoma. Dopamine is a prolactin-release inhibitory factor and disruption of the pituitary stalk leads to impaired transport of dopamine to lactotrophs resulting in increased prolactin levels. Although elevated levels of prolactin can inhibit gonadotropin secretion, a prolactinoma is generally associated with prolactin levels >2000 mU/L.

35. C. This gentleman has secondary hypothyroidism and hypogonadism in the presence of elevated prolactin levels, which are indicative of stalk compression due to a pituitary adenoma. A prolactinoma is generally associated with prolactin levels >2000 mU/L. Morbid obesity may be associated with hypogonadotrophic hypogonadism, although secondary hypothyroidism is unlikely.

Karavitaki N, Thanabalasingham G, Shore H, et al. Do the limits of serum prolactin in disconnection hyperprolactinaemia need re-definition? A study of 226 patients with histologically verified non-functioning pituitary macroadenoma. Clinical Endocrinology (Oxford), 2006; 65(4): 524–529.

36. D. The thyrotrophs and cotricotrophs are usually the last cell lines to be involved in a patient with NFPA (in contrast to relatively earlier involvement of these cell lines in patients with post-partum hypophysitis).

Melmed S. The pituitary (3rd edn). Academic Press/Elsevier, 2011.

37. C. This patient has a NFPA with elevated prolactin levels due to pituitary stalk compression. She has extensive cavernous sinus involvement due to the tumour as a result surgical treatment with conventional approach (trans-sphenoidal) is unlikely to be successful. Stereotactic gamma knife radio-surgery is a useful treatment modality in such clinical scenarios, although its availability is still quite limited.

Sheehan J, Starke R, Mathieu D, et al. Gamma knife radiosurgery for the management of nonfunctioning pituitary adenomas: a multicenter study. Journal of Neurosurgery, 2013; 119(2): 446–456.

38. B. The definitive indication of treatment for a NFPA is optic chiasm compression. Tumour size and anterior pituitary hormone dysfunction are not definitive indications for elective surgery. In a functioning pituitary adenoma (GH/ACTH/TSH/FSH) surgery remains the treatment of choice except for prolactinomas, which achieve a high cure rate with medical management (cabergoline, bromocriptine, quinagolide).

Molitch M. Nonfunctioning pituitary tumors and pituitary incidentalomas. Endocrinology Metabolism Clinic North America, 2008; 37(1): 151–171, xi.

39. C. In view of a non-functioning pituitary macroadenoma compressing optic chiasm and leading to visual field defects, the patient needs to be referred to neurosurgeons for an elective trans-sphenoidal surgery. His biochemical results are consistent with secondary hypogonadism and hypothyroidism. In a compressive pituitary adenoma, somatotrophs and gonadotrophs are the first cell lines to be affected with thyrotrophs and corticotrophs involvement at later stages.

Fernandez A, Karavitaki N, Wass JA. Prevalence of pituitary adenomas: a community-based, cross-sectional study in Banbury (Oxfordshire, UK). Clinical Endocrinology (Oxford), 2010; 72(3): 377.

Ferrante E, Ferraroni M, Castrignano T, et al. Non-functioning pituitary adenoma database: a useful resource to improve the clinical management of pituitary tumors. European Journal of Endocrinology, 2006; 155(6): 823–829.

Karavitaki N, Thanabalasingham G, Shore H, et al. Do the limits of serum prolactin in disconnection hyperprolactinaemia need re-definition? A study of 226 patients with histologically verified non-functioning pituitary macroadenoma. Clinical Endocrinology (Oxford), 2006; 65(4): 524–529.

40. B. This patient has an elevated oestradiol level in the presence of high FSH and low LH levels, together with the presence of pituitary macroadenoma on MRI pituitary, suggestive of diagnosis of a gonadotropin (FSH) secretory adenoma. It is an extremely rare tumour, and can present with enlarged ovaries and menstrual irregularities, and may initially be erroneously labelled as polycystic ovarian syndrome. The oestrogen levels may be high or within normal range. LH levels are usually suppressed. The treatment remains elective surgery to remove the pituitary adenoma.

Kajitani T, Liu S, Maruyama T, et al. Analysis of serum FSH bioactivity in a patient with an FSH-secreting pituitary microadenoma and multicystic ovaries: a case report. Human Reproduction, 2008; 23(2): 435–439.

Shimon I, Rubinek T, Bar-Hava I, et al. Ovarian hyperstimulation without elevated serum estradiol associated with pure follicle-stimulating hormone-secreting pituitary adenoma. J Clinical Endocrinology and Metabolism, 2001; 86: 3635–3640.

41. C. TSH-secreting tumours are rare causes of thyrotoxicosis and comprise 0.5–1% of all pituitary adenoma. These tumours need to be distinguished from thyroid hormone resistance syndromes, which present with similar TFT results (elevated or inappropriately normal TSH levels, in the presence of raised FT4 and FT3). TSHomas are characterized by a raised α subunit/TSH ratio >1, usually a macroadenoma on MRI pituitary, and a lack of elevation of TSH after a TRH stimulation test. A family history of thyroid dysfunction is more commonly seen in patients with thyroid hormone resistance.

42. A. The presence of inappropriately normal or elevated TSH levels in the presence of elevated T3 and T4 levels is indicative of either a TSH-secreting pituitary adenoma or the presence of thyroid hormone resistance. Rarely, such a biochemical profile is a result of presence of heterophile antibodies leading to spurious results.

TSH-secreting tumours usually present with features of mild thyrotoxicosis and goitre. The TSH α subunit secretion is increased in such tumours and is used to distinguish from thyroid hormone resistance. A molar ratio of α subunit to TSH of >5.7 is considered diagnostic in such cases. A TRH stimulation test can occasionally be used to distinguish between the two conditions, but is hardly performed these days. In contrast thyroid hormone resistance can either be generalized, selective pituitary, or selective peripheral resistance to hormone action. Most of the resistance syndromes are familial in origin. Patients are generally clinically euthyroid, except in cases of pituitary resistance to thyroid hormone. The mutation is usually at thyroid hormone receptor level.

Kienitz T, Quinkler M, Strasburger C, et al. Long-term management in five cases of TSH-secreting pituitary adenomas: a single center study and review of the literature. European Journal of Endocrinology, 2007; 157: 39–46.

Socin H, Chanson P, Delemer B, et al. The changing spectrum of TSH-secreting pituitary adenomas: diagnosis and management in 43 patients. European Journal of Endocrinology, 2003; 148: 433–442.

43. C. The main differential diagnosis for elevated FT4 and FT3 levels in the presence of a high or inappropriately normal TSH levels include a TSHoma and thyroid hormone resistance syndrome. An elevated α unit to TSH ratio is suggestive of a diagnosis of TSHoma. These are rare pituitary tumours with an incidence varying from 0.5 to 1% of all pituitary tumours. There is no response of TSH on TRH injection. Most of these patients receive anti-thyroid treatment, initially due to an erroneous diagnosis of hyperthyroidism. The TSHomas, due to its insidious onset and delay in diagnosis, are generally macroadenomas. Surgical treatment remains the treatment of choice. Octreotide therapy is the medical treatment in patients who are unresponsive to surgical therapy or who are deemed unfit for an operation.

Kienitz T, Quinkler M, Strasburger C, et al. Long-term management in five cases of TSH-secreting pituitary adenomas: a single center study and review of the literature. European Journal of Endocrinology 2007; 157: 39–46.

Socin H, Chanson P, Delemer B, et al. The changing spectrum of TSH-secreting pituitary adenomas: diagnosis and management in 43 patients. European Journal of Endocrinology, 2003; 148: 433–442.

44. A. Gonadotropins are the commonest cells of origin for NPFA on immunocytochemical staining. Most of these tumours synthesize and secrete glycoprotein hormones and/or free α or β subunits. In a NFPA the gonadotropin subunits are either secreted in low levels to have any clinical/functional significance or biologically inert at gonadal level.

Melmed S. The pituitary (3rd edn). Academic Press/Elsevier, 2011.

45. A. With the advent of radiological imaging techniques, the incidence and prevalence of pituitary incidentaloma (PI) is increasing. The prevalence of micro-incidentaloma (size <10 mm) and macro-incidentaloma (size 10 mm or greater) has been quoted between 5–30% and 0.1–0.25%, respectively, based on modality used for scanning.

According to the guidelines (2011) from Endocrine Society, patients with pituitary incidentaloma should undergo a complete history-taking and physical examination to evaluate for hormone over/under-secretion, together with laboratory evaluation of anterior pituitary hormone function test. This is based on fact that there is a high prevalence of subclinical disease, even in asymptomatic patients. A formal visual field assessment is recommended only in patients with visual field defects or a tumour compressing optic nerve or chiasm on initial radiology.

Freda PU, Beckers AM, Katznelson L, et al. Pituitary incidentaloma: an Endocrine Society clinical practice guideline. Journal of Clinical Endocrinology & Metabolism, 2011; 96(4): 894–904.

46. C. According to the Endocrine Society guidelines (2011), in patients with a pituitary micro-incidentaloma, a MRI of the pituitary gland should be repeated after 1 year (after 6 months in patients with a macro-incidentaloma). If the repeat scan does not show any interval change in the size of the tumour, then subsequent scans should be organized every 1–2 years for the first 3 years and less frequently thereafter. In patients with macro-incidentaloma, yearly scans should be arranged for the first 3 years after initial diagnosis.

In a patient with micro-incidentaloma a repeat anterior pituitary hormone profile is not routinely indicated. Anterior pituitary hormone profile should be repeated in the patients displaying features of hormone deficiency/excess based on history and examination, or if there is an increase in size of the tumour on repeat radiological investigations.

Freda PU, Beckers AM, Katznelson L, et al. Pituitary incidentaloma: an Endocrine Society clinical practice guideline. Journal of Clinical Endocrinology & Metabolism, 2011; 96(4): 894–904.

47. B. The indications for surgery in patients with PI include:
- The presence of a visual field defect.
- A lesion compressing the optic nerve or chiasm.
- Ophthalmoplegia secondary to PI.
- Pituitary apoplexy with severe visual disturbance.
- Functional tumours (ACTH, GH-secreting).

Freda PU, Beckers AM, Katznelson L, et al. Pituitary incidentaloma: an Endocrine Society clinical practice guideline. Journal of Clinical Endocrinology & Metabolism, 2011; 96(4): 894–904.

48. C. This boy has GH deficiency as a post-operative complication of craniopharyngioma resection as evidenced by delayed growth and biochemistry results. He will require 0.15–0.3 mg daily subcutaneous GH injections and the dose titration is based on IGF-1 levels (to a maximum of 1 mg/day). The main side effects associated with GH injections include fluid retention, myalgia, arthralgia, and benign intracranial hypertension. It is contraindicated in the presence of any active malignancy in the body.

Price D and Jonsson P. Effect of growth hormone treatment in children with craniopharyngioma with reference to the KIGS (Kabi International Growth Study) database. Acta Paediatrica, 1996; 417(Suppl.): 83–85.

Yuen K, Koltowska-Haggstrom M, Cook D, et al. Clinical characteristics and effects of GH replacement therapy in adults with childhood-onset craniopharyngioma compared with those in adults with other causes of childhood-onset hypothalamic-pituitary dysfunction. European Journal of Endocrinology, 2013; 169(4): 511–519.

49. A. Craniopharyngiomas are characterized by presence of an enhancing suprasellar mass, which may be cystic, and show calcification on CT scan. These tumours may lead to the development of hormonal deficiencies or may present with local pressure effects. The cysts within the tumour are filled with protein and/or cholesterol, which are usually demonstrated as a T1 high-intensity signal on MRI and described as showing a motor oil-like appearance.

Muller HL. Diagnostics, Treatment and Follow-Up in Craniopharyngioma. Frontiers in Endocrinology (Lausanne), 2011; 2: 70.

Zacharia B, Bruce S, Goldstein H, et al. Incidence, treatment and survival of patients with craniopharyngioma in the surveillance, epidemiology and end results program. Neuro-Oncology, 2012; 14(8): 1070–1078.

50. B. Lymphocytic hypophysitis is most commonly seen in women during pregnancy or the post-partum period. It is believed to be an inflammatory/autoimmune disease involving the pituitary gland and its stalk. The presenting symptoms include headache and features of hypopituitarism, such as lethargy, amenorrhoea, polydipsia, and polyuria. In contrast to pituitary adenoma, there is an early involvement of corticotrophs and thyrotrophs.

The pituitary gland may be enlarged, leading to optic chiasm compression. MRI may demonstrate a sellar homogeneous mass, together with thickening of stalk. The diagnosis is established on histology, which shows diffuse lymphocytic infiltration. Medical management usually involves supportive therapy and the use of steroids.

Bellastella A, Bizzarro A, Coronella C, et al. Lymphocytic hypophysitis: a rare or underestimated disease? European Journal of Endocrinology, 2003; 149: 363–376.

51. C. He needs to be started on hydrocortisone replacement therapy, based on low post-operative cortisol levels. His anterior pituitary hormone function should be re-assessed 6 weeks post-operatively, together with a formal short synacthen test (after withholding the evening dose of hydrocortisone). A repeat MRI of the pituitary should be arranged in 6–8 weeks time to assess for residual tumour.

52. E. Polydipsia and polyuria during the post-operative period (after trans-sphenoidal surgery) is commonly seen secondary to a transient cranial diabetes insipidus. The input/output of patients should be monitored closely. Patients may need desmopressin therapy (intranasally 10–40 μg/day or orally 200–400 μg/day) if symptoms persist and diagnosis is confirmed based on serum and urine osmolality measurement. There is an increased association of transient diabetes insipidus (DI) with intra-operative CSF leak, macroadenoma, craniopharyngioma and Rathke cleft cyst.

Hensen J, Henig A, Fahlbusch R, et al. Prevalence, predictors and patterns of postoperative polyuria and hyponatraemia in the immediate course after transsphenoidal surgery for pituitary adenomas. Clinical Endocrinology (Oxford), 1999; 50(4): 431–439.

Nemergut E, Zuo Z, Jane J and Laws E. Predictors of diabetes insipidus after transsphenoidal surgery: a review of 881 patients. Journal of Neurosurgery. 2005; 103(3): 448–454.

53. A. β transferrin is an isoform of transferrin which is almost exclusively found in CSF. As it is not present in blood, mucus or tears, it is considered a specific marker of CSF. It is a useful assay in patients where CSF leakage is suspected during the post-operative period.

Chan D, Poon W, Chiu P, et al. How useful is glucose detection in diagnosing cerebrospinal fluid leak? The rational use of CT and Beta-2 transferrin assay in detection of cerebrospinal fluid fistula. Asian Journal of Surgery, 2004; 27(1): 39–42.

54. B. Octreotide therapy is associated with the development of gall stones and a decrease in gall bladder contractility. Tumour size reduction of >20% is seen in 75% patients treated with somatostatin analogues. Gastrointestinal side effects, such as anorexia, nausea, vomiting, flatulence, and diarrhoea, are commonly seen. Post-prandial glucose tolerance may be impaired, although hypoglycaemia has also been reported.

Melmed S, Casanueva F, Klibanski A, et al. A consensus on criteria for cure of acromegaly, Journal of Clinical Endocrinology & Metabolism, 2010; 95(7): 3141–3148.

55. E. Pasireotide (SOM 230) is a novel somatostatin analogue that acts on SSTR subtypes 2, 3, and 5, as compared with octreotide, which has selective affinity for SSTR2. It leads to a decrease in IGF-1 and GH levels, although there is an increased risk of development of gall stones due to the alteration of bile composition and reduced gall bladder wall contractility. Somatostatin analogues have a direct inhibitory effect on insulin secretion, which may lead to a worsening of glycaemic control in patients with diabetes or the development of impaired glucose tolerance in individuals without diabetes.

Petersenn S, Farrall A, Block C, et al. Long-term efficacy and safety of subcutaneous pasireotide in acromegaly: results from an open-ended, multicenter, Phase II extension study. Pituitary, 2014; 17: 132–140.

56. A. The water deprivation test involves a serial measurement (2-hourly) of serum and urine osmolality, together with body weight for a period of 6–8 hours in patients suspected to have DI. A serum osmolality of >290 mOsmol/Kg, together with urine osmolality of <300 mOsmol/Kg is suggestive of DI. The diagnosis of central DI is confirmed if there is an increase in urine osmolality >750 mOsmol/Kg after desmopressin. In patients with nephrogenic DI, there is a lack of response to desmopressin. In contrast, patients with psychogenic polydipsia have a low serum osmolality along with appropriate increase in urine osmolality with water deprivation.

In clinical practice, the water deprivation test may yield equivocal results due to partial cranial DI or inability to concentrate urine due to long standing history of psychogenic polydipsia.

Diederich S, Eckmanns T, Exner P, et al. Differential diagnosis of polyuric/polydipsic syndromes with the aid of urinary vasopressin measurement in adults. Clinical Endocrinology (Oxford), 2001; 54(5): 665.

57. B. The presence of Type 1 DM, visual impairment (probably secondary to optic atrophy) and DI-based water deprivation test results is consistent with a diagnosis of Wolfram syndrome (DIDMOAD). This condition has an autosomal recessive mode of inheritance. Diabetes and optic atrophy are usually the first manifestations (presenting in the 1st and 2nd decades) followed by diabetes insipidus (present in 70–80%) and deafness (present in 65–70%) in the 2nd and 3rd decades. The patients may develop features of hypogonadism and progressive neurological disorders, such as ataxia and myoclonus.

Barrett T, Bundey S, and Macleod A. Neurodegeneration and diabetes: UK nationwide study of Wolfram (DIDMOAD) syndrome. Lancet, 1995; 346(8988): 1458–1463.

58. B. Germinomas are a rare and heterogeneous group of intracranial tumours. These tumours are most commonly seen in children/young adults, and may present with symptoms of anterior pituitary dysfunction and/or diabetes insipidus. The diagnosis of DI in young adults, together with a mass lesion on radiological imaging should warrant the measurement of serum/CSF β-hCG and α-foetoprotein levels. The definitive diagnosis is based on histological analysis. Immunostaining with markers like NANOG (which is a homeodomain transcription factor) is sensitive, as well as specific for the diagnosis of germinoma and is considered a better marker than OCT3/4, SOX 2. These tumours are sensitive to radiotherapy, although they may need adjuvant chemotherapy.

Gutenberg A, Bell J, Lupi I, et al. Pituitary and systemic autoimmunity in a case of intrasellar germinoma. Pituitary, 2011; 14: 388–394.

Santagata S, Hornick J, and Ligon K. Comparative analysis of germ cell transcription factors in CNS germinoma reveals diagnostic utility of NANOG. American Journal of Surgical Pathology, 2006; 30(12): 1613–1618.

59. A. The symptoms associated with excess GH/IGF-1 secretion, as seen in acromegaly, includes the coarsening of facial features, an increase in ring/shoe size, prognathism, increased sweating, macroglossia, wide spacing of teeth, and enlargement of extremities. A random serum IGF-1 level measurement is useful for diagnosis (and monitoring of response after therapeutic intervention). Due to variation in GH secretion on a day-to-day basis, a random GH hormone measurement is of limited clinical use. OGTT is a useful test to help establish the underlying diagnosis of acromegaly. It is performed by the consumption of 75 g of oral glucose, followed by half-hourly GH measurement (for 2 hours). A serum GH value <1 ng/mL after OGTT is considered normal, with a serum GH nadir value of 0.3 ng/mL believed to increase the sensitivity of the test. In patients with clinical and biochemical evidence of excess GH secretion, MRI pituitary should be arranged to identify GH-secreting adenoma.

Katznelson L, Atkinson JL, Cook DM, et al. American Association of Clinical Endocrinologists medical guidelines for clinical practice for the diagnosis and management of acromegaly—2011 update. Endocrine Practice, 2011; 17(Suppl. 4).

60. A. This case demonstrates co-secretion of GH and prolactin by a pituitary adenoma. Cabergoline therapy can be started immediately to treat hyperprolactinaemia in the outpatient setting and may help shrinkage of the tumour while she awaits elective trans-sphenoidal surgery.

Freda P, Reyes C, Nuruzzaman A, et al. Cabergoline therapy of growth hormone & growth hormone/prolactin secreting pituitary tumors. Pituitary, 2004; 7(1): 21–30.

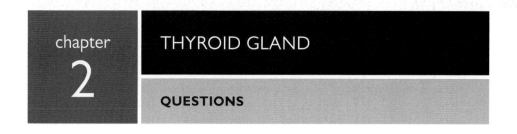

1. During embryological development, the thyroid gland originates from the floor of the pharynx as an outpouching. Microscopically, the gland is composed of a series of follicles that synthesize thyroglobulin (Tg) and parafollicular (C cells), which secrete calcitonin during adult life.

    The embryological origin for the parafollicular cells of thyroid is from which one of the following source?

    A. Base of the tongue
    B. Endoderm of the floor of pharynx
    C. Foramen caecum
    D. Lateral pharyngeal pouches
    E. Neural crest

2. Thyroid hormones are transported in serum, bound to carrier proteins such as thyroxine-binding globulin (TBG), thyroxine-binding pre-albumin (TBPA) and albumin. TBG comprises a single polypeptide chain (containing four carbohydrate chains), and is the major transporter of thyroid hormones.

    Which one of the following is associated with an increase in TBG levels?

    A. Active acromegaly
    B. Anabolic steroids
    C. Androgens
    D. Chronic liver disease
    E. Tamoxifen

3. **A 17-year-old girl was incidentally detected to have abnormal thyroid function test (TFT) results, as part of routine tests to ascertain the cause of her tiredness. She denied any weight gain, menstrual irregularity, cold intolerance, or constipation. She had a strong family history of thyroid dysfunction with her two elder brothers and maternal uncles suffering from abnormal thyroid function, although none received any medications. On examination, she had mild tremors in her hands and a pulse rate of 76 beats/minute with rest of the general physical and systemic examination being unremarkable.**

    ```
    TFT results:
      free T4   24.4 pmol/L (11.5-19.7)
      free T3   7.8 pmol/L (3.5-6.5)
      TSH       7.2 mU/L (0.35-5.5)
    ```

    Which one of the following is the most likely diagnosis based on her clinical profile?

    A. Pregnancy
    B. Prolactinoma
    C. Subclinical hyperthyroidism
    D. Subclinical hypothyroidism
    E. Thyroid hormone resistance

4. **A 17-year-old girl was incidentally detected to have abnormal thyroid function test results as a part of her routine tests to ascertain the cause of her tiredness. She denied any weight gain, menstrual irregularity, cold intolerance or constipation. She had a strong family history of thyroid dysfunction with her 2 elder brothers and maternal uncles suffering from abnormal thyroid function although none received any medications.**

    On examination, she had mild tremors in the hands, pulse rate of 76 beats/minute with rest of the general physical and systemic examination being normal.

    ```
    Her TFT results were as shown:
      free T4   24.4 pmol/L (11.5-19.7)
      free T3   7.8 pmol/L (3.5-6.5)
      TSH       7.2 mU/L (0.35-5.5)
    ```

    Genetic analysis confirmed the diagnosis of thyroid hormone resistance syndrome.

    Which one of the following is most commonly associated with thyroid hormone resistance syndrome?

    A. Heterozygous mutation of both TRα and TRβ gene
    B. Heterozygous mutation of TRα gene
    C. Heterozygous mutation of TRβ gene
    D. Homozygous mutation of TRα gene
    E. Homozygous mutation of TRβ gene

5. **TSH synthesis and secretion is mainly influenced by serum levels of thyroid hormones (T4 and T3) and, to a certain extent, by a few hormones and drugs.**

   Which one of the following medications/hormones stimulates the release of TSH?

   A. Arginine-vasopressin
   B. Dopamine agonists
   C. Glucocorticoids
   D. Growth hormone
   E. Somatostatin

6. **TSH controls the thyroid cell growth and hormone synthesis by binding to specific TSH receptor (TSH-R).**

   Which one of the following is a correct description for TSH-R?

   A. Intra-cytoplasmic receptor
   B. Nuclear receptor
   C. Peptide receptor
   D. Steroid type receptor
   E. Trans-membrane G protein coupled receptor

7. **Thyroid follicle cells synthesize thyroglobulin, which is comprised of tyrosyl residues, carbohydrates, and iodide.**

   Which one of the following conditions is associated with decreased Tg levels?

   A. Graves' disease (GD)
   B. Hyperthyroidism
   C. Sub-acute thyroiditis
   D. Thyrotoxicosis factitia
   E. Untreated differentiated thyroid cancers

8. **A 70-year-old man was admitted to the intensive care unit with features of septicaemia due to community-acquired pneumonia. His blood tests showed thyroid dysfunction that was attributed to a non-thyroidal illness or sick euthyroid state.**

   Which one of the following is the typical pattern of thyroid dysfunction seen in a sick euthyroid illness?

   A. Elevated levels of T3 and T4; low levels of reverse T3
   B. Elevated levels of T3, T4, and reverse T3
   C. Low levels of T3 and T4; elevated levels of reverse T3
   D. Low levels of T3 and T4; normal of reverse T3
   E. Low levels of T3, T4, and reverse T3

9. Thyroid hormone signalling can alter at individual tissue level, based on activation or inactivation of thyroid hormone by the process of de-iodination. Three different deiodinase enzymes are known to exist and play a part in influencing thyroid hormone signalling at tissue level.

    Which one of the following correctly describes the commonest 5' deiodinase enzyme present in neurons and its role?

    A. Type 1 deiodinase leading to decreased T3
    B. Type 1 deiodinase leading to increased T3
    C. Type 2 deiodinase leading to decreased T3
    D. Type 2 deiodinase leading to increased T3
    E. Type 3 deiodinase leading to increased T3

10. Which one of the following medications is associated with an increase in serum-free thyroid hormone levels?

    A. Cholestyramine
    B. Heparin
    C. Iron preparations
    D. Lithium
    E. Oestrogen

11. A 28-year-old woman presented to the thyroid clinic with a lump in her neck that was first noticed by her about 4 weeks ago. On examination, a 2-cm left-sided thyroid nodule was palpable. The histopathology report of the fine needle aspiration cytology confirmed the presence of Thy3 cytology.

    Which one of the following is the most appropriate management approach for a Thy3 cytology, based on British Thyroid Association (BTA) guidelines (2007)?

    A. Discharge from follow-up
    B. Left lobectomy
    C. Radio-iodine ablation
    D. Repeat fine needle aspiration cytology (FNAC) in 3–6 months
    E. Total thyroidectomy

12. A 60-year-old woman was referred by her GP to the thyroid clinic with a painless lump in the neck first noticed about 3 months ago. On examination, a 1.5-cm firm thyroid nodule was palpable. The histopathology report of the fine needle aspiration cytology confirmed the presence of Thy2 cytology.

    Which one of the following is the correct description of Thy2 cytology?

    A. Follicular adenoma
    B. Follicular carcinoma
    C. Non-diagnostic test
    D. Non-neoplastic lesion
    E. Suspicious malignancy

13. **A 45-year-old man of Indian sub-continent origin presented to the clinic with symptoms of malaise, weight gain, and cold intolerance. He had a past medical history of primary autoimmune hypothyroidism and had been taking thyroxine (100 µg/day) for the last 5 years. He had been reviewed in a respiratory clinic 6 weeks earlier and diagnosed with pulmonary tuberculosis. As a result, he was initiated on a combination chemotherapy regimen for tuberculosis, comprising isoniazid, rifampicin, ethambutol, and pyrazinamide.**

```
TFT's results:
   free T4             10.2 pmol/L (11.5-22.7)
   TSH                 10.4 mU/L (0.35-5.5)
   Anti-TPO antibody   Positive
```

Which one of the following is the most likely explanation for his symptoms and biochemistry results?

A. Flare-up of autoimmune activity with tuberculosis
B. Thyroxine interaction with ethambutol
C. Thyroxine interaction with isoniazid
D. Thyroxine interaction with rifampicin
E. Poor compliance

14. **A 44-year-old woman presented to her GP with occasional episodes of palpitations and flushing lasting for few minutes. These episodes had no obvious precipitating factor and were not associated with any chest pain or tightness. On examination, she had resting tremors, a pulse rate of 84 beats/minute with regular rhythm. Her general physical and systemic examination was unremarkable.**

```
Investigations:
   free T4                 20.2 pmol/L (11.5-22.7)
   TSH                     0.25 mU/L (0.35-5.5)
   TSH receptor antibody   negative
```

Which one of the following is the most appropriate management approach, based on her clinical profile and test results?

A. Commence on carbimazole
B. Commence on β-blockers only
C. Observe and monitor TFTs
D. Radioactive iodine ablation (RAIA)
E. Arrange a thyroid uptake scan

15. **A 40-year-old woman presented to her GP with general lethargy and difficulty in sleeping. She was not on any regular drug replacement and there was no family history of thyroid disease. Her general physical and systemic examination was unremarkable.**

    ```
    TFT results:
      free T4   23.8 pmol/L  (11.5-19.7)
      free T3   8.8 pmol/L   (3.5-6.5)
      TSH       5.8 mU/L      (0.35-5.5)
    ```

    Which one of the following is the most appropriate next step in her management?

    A. Commence carbimazole
    B. Commence thyroxine
    C. Consider assay interference
    D. Genetic tests for thyroid hormone resistance
    E. Urgent MRI pituitary

16. **A 66-year-old farmer was incidentally detected to have abnormal thyroid function while he was hospitalized for a pulmonary embolism and undergoing anti-coagulation therapy with low molecular weight heparin.**

    ```
    TFT results:
      free T4   22.5 pmol/L  (11.5-19.7)
      free T3   6.8 pmol/L   (3.5-6.5)
      TSH       4.8 mU/L      (0.35-5.5)
    ```

    Which one of the following is the most appropriate step in his immediate management?

    A. Commence carbimazole
    B. Consider RAI
    C. Observe
    D. Thyroid uptake scan
    E. Urgent MRI pituitary

17. **A 32-year-old woman was admitted to the medical assessment unit with nausea, vomiting, and dehydration. She also complained of intermittent headaches and visual blurring.**

    ```
    TFT results:
      FT3   7.1 pmol/L  (3.5-6.5)
      FT4   21.3 pmol/L  (11.5-19.7)
      TSH   4.1 mu/L     (0.35-5.5)
    ```

    Which one of the following test may be useful to diagnose TSHoma?

    A. A 3-mm lesion in the pituitary on MRI
    B. Blunted or absent response to TRH stimulation
    C. Decreased α subunit/TSH molar ratio
    D. Low to normal level of SHBG
    E. Negative gene sequencing for *THRB* gene

18. **A 35-year-old woman presented to her GP with increasing anxiety, palpitations, weight loss, and irregular menstrual periods. On examination, she had bilateral tremors, proptosis, and a palpable small goitre.**

```
TFT results:
   free T4                  27.2 pmol/L (11.5-22.7)
   TSH                      <0.01 mU/L (0.35-5.5)
   TSH receptor antibody    Positive
   anti-TPO antibody        Positive
```

What percentage of patients with Graves' disease demonstrates a positive anti-thyroid peroxidase (anti-TPO) antibody status?

A. <5%

B. 15–20%

C. 40–50%

D. 70–80%

E. 95–100%

19. **A 22-year-old man presented to his GP with weight gain, lethargy, and cold intolerance. He was on thyroxine (125 µg) tablets for primary autoimmune hypothyroidism. He was also taking insulin (basal-bolus regimen) for Type 1 DM, diagnosed when he was 11 years old.**

```
TFT results:
   free T4   22.5 pmol/L (11.5-22.7)
   free T3   6.4 pmol/L (3.5-6.5)
   TSH       8.2 mU/L (0.35-5.5)
```

Which one of the following is the most appropriate management approach in his clinical scenario?

A. Counselling regarding compliance with therapy

B. Increase thyroxine dose

C. Reduce thyroxine dose

D. Repeat TFT's in 6–8 weeks

E. Switch to liothyronine (T3)

20. **Which one of the following body fluids has a 50-fold lower concentration of thyroid hormones and metabolites levels compared with serum?**

A. Breast milk

B. CSF

C. Saliva

D. Tissue fluid

E. Urine

21. **A 70-year-old retired teacher presented to the thyroid clinic with a 3-month history of anxiety, recurrent bouts of palpitations, and increased sweating. He had a past medical history of hypertension and atrial fibrillation. He was taking amiodarone, lisinopril, and bisoprolol therapy.**

```
Investigations:
   TSH                      <0.01 mU/L (0.35-5.5)
   free T4                  30.5 pmol/L (11.5-22.7)
   anti-TPO antibodies      positive
   TSH receptor antibodies  negative
```

He underwent a radioactive iodine uptake (RAIU) scan (see Figure 2.1).

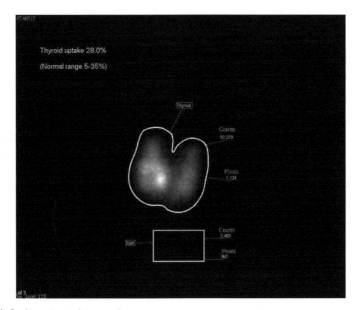

Figure 2.1 Radioactive iodine uptake scan

Reproduced with permission from Dr Nimit Goyal, Consultant Radiologist, Royal Gwent Hospital, Newport, UK

Which one of the following is the most appropriate therapeutic option for his further management?

A. Carbimazole

B. Prednisolone

C. Propanolol

D. RAIA

E. Subtotal thyroidectomy

22. **A 63-year-old woman presented to her GP with palpitations and weight loss. She had background medical history of intractable atrial fibrillation (AF) for which she was under cardiology follow-up, and taking bisoprolol and amiodarone therapy. On examination, she had bilateral tremors, no eye signs of Graves' orbitopathy (GO), and AF with a ventricular rate of 90–100 beats/minute.**

```
TFT results:
  TSH                        <0.01 mU/L (0.35-5.5)
  free T4                    29.9 pmol/L (11.5-22.7)
  TSH receptor antibodies    negative
  thyroid uptake scan        <1% uptake
```

Which one of the following is the most appropriate management option for her?

A. Carbimazole

B. Prednisolone

C. Radio-iodine ablation

D. Stop amiodarone

E. Subtotal thyroidectomy

23. **A woman who was 10 weeks pregnant presented with nausea, vomiting, and palpitations for 2 weeks. She had a family history of thyroid dysfunction, with her elder sister and mother having undergone RAIA therapy for an overactive thyroid gland. On examination, she was dehydrated with tachycardia and bilateral tremors. She also had proptosis and a small palpable goitre with an audible bruit.**

```
TFT results:
  free T4   40.5 pmol/L (11.5-22.7)
  free T3   15.4 pmol/L (3.5-6.5)
  TSH       <0.01 mU/L (0.35-5.5)
```

Which one of the following investigations will be most useful to plan her further management?

A. β-hCG levels

B. FNAC thyroid nodule

C. Thyroid ultrasound

D. Thyroid uptake scan

E. TSH receptor antibody

24. **A woman who was 12 weeks pregnant presented with nausea, vomiting, and palpitations for 2 weeks. She had a family history of thyroid dysfunction with her elder sister and mother having undergone RAI therapy for an overactive thyroid gland. On examination, she was dehydrated with tachycardia and bilateral tremors. She also had proptosis and a small palpable goitre with an audible bruit.**

```
TFT results:
   free T4                40.5 pmol/L (11.5-22.7)
   free T3                15.4 pmol/L (3.5-6.5)
   TSH                    <0.01 mU/L (0.35-5.5)
   TSH receptor antibody  positive
```

Which one of the following is the most appropriate therapeutic approach in her case?

A. Carbimazole
B. Observe
C. Propanolol
D. RAIA
E. Subtotal thyroidectomy

25. **A 30-year-old woman who was 8 weeks pregnant presented to the joint antenatal-endocrine clinic, with mild early morning nausea and tiredness. She was diagnosed with primary autoimmune hypothyroidism about 5 years ago and was taking thyroxine (100 μg od) therapy. On examination, she was clinically euthyroid and systemically well.**

```
TFT results:
   free T4  14.5 pmol/L (11.5-22.7)
   free T3  4.2 pmol/L (3.5-6.5)
   TSH      10.5 mU/L (0.35-5.5)
```

Which one of the following is the most appropriate management approach in her clinical scenario?

A. Check anti-TPO antibodies
B. Check compliance
C. Increase thyroxine dose
D. Observe and repeat TFTs in 4–6 weeks
E. Reduce thyroxine dose

26. **A 24-year-old woman who was 10 weeks pregnant presented to the joint antenatal-endocrine clinic with symptoms of nausea and early morning sickness. On examination, she had pulse rate of 78 beats/minute with no clinical features of hyperthyroidism.**

```
TFTs results:
   Free T4   19.9 pmol/L  (11.5-22.7)
   TSH        0.8 mU/L  (0.35-5.5)
```

Which one of the following is the correct management approach in her clinical scenario?

A. Arrange RAI
B. Check TSH receptor antibodies
C. Start carbimazole
D. Sub-total thyroidectomy in 2nd trimester
E. Thyroid uptake scan

27. **A 24-year-old woman was admitted to the assessment unit with nausea, recurrent vomiting, and features of dehydration. She was 8 weeks pregnant, and denied any abdominal pain or vaginal discharge. On examination, she was dehydrated with a heart rate of 88/minute and blood pressure of 100/70 mmHg. The rest of her general physical and systemic examination was unremarkable.**

```
TFT results:
   free T4                  25.5 pmol/L  (11.5-22.7)
   free T3                  7.2 pmol/L  (3.5-6.5)
   TSH                      0.15 mU/L  (0.35-5.5)
   TSH receptor antibodies  negative
```

Which one of the following is the most appropriate management approach for her thyroid dysfunction?

A. Carbimazole
B. Observation
C. Propanolol
D. Propylthiouracil
E. Thyroidectomy

28. **A 27-year-old woman presented to her GP with anxiety, palpitations, and increased sweating. She was 8 weeks post-partum and not on any medications. On examination, she had bilateral tremors and a pulse rate of 96 beats/minute, with no eye signs of Graves' disease or goitre.**

    ```
    TFT results:
       free T4                   22.5 pmol/L (11.5-22.7)
       TSH                       <0.18 mU/L (0.35-5.5)
       TSH receptor antibodies   negative
    ```

    Which one of the following is the most appropriate management approach in her case?

    A. Carbimazole

    B. Propanolol

    C. Propylthiouracil

    D. RAIA

    E. Subtotal thyroidectomy

29. **A 35-year-old woman presented to thyroid clinic with features of malaise, lethargy, and weight gain 6 months after her delivery. On examination, she had a pulse rate of 60 beats/minute, and cold, dry skin, although systemic examination was unremarkable.**

    ```
    TFT results:
       free T4     5.8 pmol/L (11.5-22.7)
       TSH         14.0 mU/L (0.35-5.5)
    ```

    The presence of which one of the following clinical features has minimal (or no) impact on the risk of development of post-partum thyroiditis?

    A. Family history of thyroid dysfunction

    B. Lymphoma

    C. Positive anti-TPO antibody titre

    D. Previous post-partum thyroiditis

    E. Type I DM

30. **A 28-year-old woman was reviewed in the joint antenatal-endocrine clinic during a routine appointment. She was 10 weeks pregnant and asymptomatic, apart from having mild early morning sickness. She had a strong family history of thyroid dysfunction and was keen to explore her risk of developing the same during pregnancy or post-partum period.**

    Which one of the following subgroup of women requires targeted case-finding during pregnancy?

    A. Family history of auto-immune thyroid disease

    B. Infertility

    C. Presence of goitre

    D. Previous miscarriage

    E. All of the above

31. **A 42-year-old bank manager presented to her GP with a 6-week history of feeling generally unwell and with a double vision. She had also noticed redness in the white of the eye with a gritty sensation for last few months. On examination, she was apyrexial with redness of the conjunctiva, lid retraction, and a proptosis that was more marked in the left eye. Eye movements were not restricted and visual acuity on formal testing was normal. Systemic examination was unremarkable.**

```
Investigations:
  free T4                   16.5 pmol/L (11.5-22.7)
  TSH                       1.4 mU/L (0.35-5.5)
  anti-TPO antibody         Negative
  C-reactive protein (CRP)  5 mg/L (<6)
```

Which one of the following is the most likely explanation for her visual symptoms and signs?

A. Carotid-cavernous fistula
B. Closed angle glaucoma
C. Graves' orbitopathy
D. Orbital cellulitis
E. Orbital tumour

32. **A 50-year-old man with Graves' eye disease complained of eye pain and double vision on a follow-up visit in thyroid clinic. He was on a block and replacement regimen of carbimazole and thyroxine. On examination, his pulse rate was 80 beats/minute and he had bilateral proptosis with no restriction of eye movement.**

```
TFT results:
  free T4  16.5 pmol/L (11.5-22.7)
  free T3  4.4 pmol/L (3.5-6.5)
  TSH      2.8 mU/L (0.35-5.5)
```

All of the following tests are essential for assessment and management of Graves' orbitopathy (GO) except?

A. Colour vision assessment
B. Fundoscopy
C. Slit lamp examination
D. Visual acuity
E. Visual evoked potential

33. **A 38-year-old teacher, with known Graves' disease, presented to the thyroid clinic with dryness of the eyes and a gritty sensation. She was previously treated with a titrating regimen of carbimazole and had been in remission for the last 3 years. On examination, her visual acuity and eye movements were normal, with no features of corneal or conjunctival involvement.**

```
TFT results:
  free T4  15.5 pmol/L (11.5-22.7)
  TSH       1.3 mU/L (0.35-5.5)
```

Which one of the following is a useful measure in the management of patients with mild GO?

A. Acetazolamide
B. Artificial tears
C. Bumetanide
D. Systemic steroids
E. Topical steroids

34. **A 24-year-old woman presented to the thyroid clinic with symptoms of anxiety, palpitations, heat intolerance, and weight loss. She also complained of redness and grittiness of her eyes. On examination, she had conjunctival redness and chemosis with bilateral proptosis.**

```
TFT results:
  free T4                33.5 pmol/L (11.5-22.7)
  free T3                10.7 pmol/L (3.5-6.5)
  TSH                    <0.01 mU/L (0.35-5.5)
  TSH receptor antibody  positive
```

Which one of the following is used as a parameter to assess the clinical activity score (CAS) in patients with GO?

A. Eyelid erythema
B. Intra-ocular pressure
C. Level of free T3 and T4
D. Level of TSH receptor antibodies
E. Lid lag

35. **A 40-year-old woman presented to the thyroid clinic with a 6-month history of weight loss, menstrual irregularities, and increased sweating. On examination, she had bilateral tremors, a pulse rate of 120 beats/ minute and an enlarged thyroid gland. Her eye movements were restricted to the lateral gaze along with the presence of bilateral proptosis. She also had an audible bruit on auscultation of neck.**

```
TFT results:
    free T4                 44.4 pmol/L (11.5-19.7)
    free T3                 16.8 pmol/L (3.5-6.5)
    TSH                     <0.1 mU/L (0.35-5.5)
    TSH receptor antibody   strongly positive
```

Which one of the following is the first line of treatment in patients with moderate to severe active GO?

A. Orbital decompression

B. Radio-iodine ablation

C. Subtotal thyroidectomy

D. Systemic steroids

E. Topical steroids

36. **A 29-year-old beautician, diagnosed as having Graves' disease 6 weeks ago, presented to medical assessment unit with reduced vision. She was taking carbimazole (40 mg/day) and had noticed an improvement in her initial symptoms of anxiety, palpitations, and diarrhoea since the initiation of the therapy. On examination, she had bilateral proptosis, swelling of eye lids, and diminished vision in her right eye. She was reviewed by ophthalmologist and initiated on pulse dosage of methyl prednisolone therapy. Her vision showed further signs of deterioration, despite the steroid therapy.**

Which one of the following is the correct management approach in her case?

A. Botulinum toxin injection

B. Interferons

C. Orbital decompression

D. Orbital radiotherapy

E. Thyroidectomy

37. **A 48-year-old care home worker was referred to the thyroid eye clinic with double vision. She had background history of Graves' disease, which was treated with a 6-month course of block and replacement therapy about 5 years ago, and she had been in disease remission since then. After review in the thyroid eye clinic, she was told that her left eye has become 'lazy' and couple of muscles were not working properly.**

    Which one of the following are the two most commonly involved muscles in a patient with GO?

    A. Inferior and medial rectus
    B. Inferior oblique and lateral rectus
    C. Medial and lateral rectus
    D. Superior and inferior oblique
    E. Superior oblique and medial rectus

38. **A 22-year-old medical student was reviewed in the thyroid eye clinic with symptoms of double vision and blurring while she was studying for her exams. On examination, she had lid lag and bilateral proptosis, although there were no clinical features of hyperthyroidism.**

    ```
    TFT results:
        free T4                18.0 pmol/L (11.5-19.7)
        TSH                    0.6 mU/L (0.35-5.5)
        TSH receptor antibody  negative
    ```

    Which one of the following is not a characteristic histological finding in patients with GO?

    A. Eosinophilic infiltration
    B. Extra-ocular muscle oedema
    C. Fibroblast stimulation
    D. Lymphocytic infiltration
    E. Scarring of orbital tissue

39. **A 28-year-old PhD student presented to the medical clinic with symptoms of weight loss, palpitations, and menorrhagia. She had also noticed some change in the appearance of her eyes, which appear to be more swollen in the early hours of the morning.**

    On examination, she had tachycardia, bilateral resting tremors, and a small goitre. Her visual acuity was normal with no restriction in eye movements.

    Which one of the following is the earliest and commonest sign associated with GO?

    A. Conjunctival chemosis
    B. Lid lag
    C. Proptosis
    D. Restricted eye movements
    E. Upper lid retraction

40. A 49-year-old man with a background history of GD in remission, presented to the thyroid clinic with a decline in vision. Apart from the occasional episode of headache, he was well and not on any medications. On examination, he had a scleral show of 2 mm in the inferior aspect with no evidence of conjunctival redness. His visual acuity was <6/18 in his left eye (previously normal) and eye movements were normal with some new onset visual complaints.

```
TFT results:
   free T4   18.4 pmol/L (11.5-19.7)
   free T3   5.8 pmol/L (3.5-6.5)
   TSH       0.46 mU/L (0.35-5.5)
```

Which one of the following is the most appropriate management approach for this patient?

A. Carbimazole
B. MRI orbits
C. Observe
D. Oral prednisolone
E. Referral to ophthalmologist

41. A 17-year-old boy presented to thyroid clinic with a 3-month history of feeling unwell, weight loss, anxiety, and panic attacks. He also complained of redness and grittiness of eyes, with painful eye movements. On examination, he had bilateral tremors, proptosis, and lid retraction.

```
Investigations:
   free T4                30.5 pmol/L (11.5-19.7)
   free T3                9.9 pmol/L (3.5-6.5)
   TSH                    <0.01 mU/L (0.35-5.5)
   TSH receptor antibody  negative
```

Which one of the following factors is associated with increased risk for the development of severe GO?

A. Free T4 and T3 levels
B. Male sex
C. No response to thionamides
D. Smoking
E. Young age

42. **A 27-year-old man presented to the thyroid clinic with symptoms of anxiety, palpitations, heat intolerance, and weight loss. He had a background history of Graves' disease that was treated with a 6-month course of block and replacement regimen comprising of thyroxine and carbimazole about 2 years ago. He had been in disease remission since then. On examination, he had tremors, smooth goitre, and increased sweating.**

```
Investigations:
  free T4  28.2 pmol/L (11.5-19.7)
  free T3  9.0 pmol/L (3.5-6.5)
  TSH      <0.01 mU/L (0.35-5.5)
```

Based on his clinical profile, a diagnosis of relapse of Graves' disease was made, and he was counselled for elective radioiodine ablative (RAI) therapy. He was keen to know the risk of RAI on his fertility.

Which one of the following is the minimum duration during that it is advisable for the men receiving RAI not to father a child?

A. 1–2 weeks

B. 1–2 months

C. 3–4 months

D. 6–8 months

E. >1 year

43. **A 36-year-old woman presented to her primary care physician with symptoms of weight loss, restlessness, and menorrhagia. She had no family history of thyroid dysfunction. On examination, she had a pulse rate of 108 beats/minute, tremors, increased sweating, and a small goitre is palpable in neck.**

```
Investigations:
  free T4               29.7 pmol/L (11.5-19.7)
  free T3               11.0 pmol/L (3.5-6.5)
  TSH                   <0.01 mU/L (0.35-5.5)
  TSH receptor antibody negative
  RAIU scan             increased uptake showing a right-sided
                        nodule
```

She was counselled for RAIA therapy.

Which one of the following is the minimum duration during which it is advisable for the women receiving RAI to avoid conception?

A. 1–2 weeks

B. 4–6 weeks

C. 2–3 months

D. 4–6 months

E. At least 1 year

44. **A 43-year-old woman was reviewed in the thyroid clinic at a follow-up appointment 2 months after she had undergone RAI therapy treatment for recurrent GD. She complained of non-specific symptoms including lethargy and a lack of appetite.**

On examination, her heart rate was 80 beats/minute with no signs of thyroid eye disease.

```
TFT results:
   free T4   22.5 pmol/L (11.5-19.7)
   free T3   6.2 pmol/L (3.5-6.5)
   TSH       0.05 mU/L (0.35-5.5)
```

Which one of the following is the most appropriate management approach at this stage?

A. Carbimazole
B. Propanolol
C. Propylthiouracil
D. Second dose of RAI treatment
E. Repeat TFT's in 8–12 weeks time

45. **A 57-year-old women presented to the endocrine clinic with symptoms of palpitations and weight loss. She had a strong family history of breast and thyroid cancers.**

On examination, she had mild tremors in the hands, no eye signs of Graves' eye disease, and a right-sided firm thyroid nodule palpable.

```
Investigations:
   free T4                 30.5 pmol/L (11.5-19.7)
   TSH                     <0.01 mU/L (0.35-5.5)
   TSH receptor antibody   negative
   RAIU scan               >30%
```

She was counselled for RAIA therapy in view of clinical features of toxic nodular goitre. She was very anxious about her increased risk of developing cancer after RAI therapy.

Which one of the following is correct regarding the association of RAI therapy and cancer development?

A. Increased risk of head and neck carcinoma
B. Increased risk of lymphoma
C. Increased risk of medullary thyroid carcinoma
D. Increased risk of papillary thyroid carcinoma
E. No increased risk of cancers

46. **A 34-year-old nurse presented to her GP with symptoms of palpitations and anxiety. On examination, she had mild tremors and a pulse rate of 100 beats/minute. The rest of her systemic examination was unremarkable.**

    ```
    Investigations:
       free T4                    25.7 pmol/L (11.5-19.7)
       free T3                    7.8 pmol/L (3.5-6.5)
       TSH                        <0.01 mU/L (0.35-5.5)
       TSH receptor antibody      negative
       RAIU scan                  <1%
    ```

    Which one of the following is associated with a normal/increased uptake on RAIU scan?

    A. Amiodarone-induced thyroiditis
    B. Factitious ingestion of thyroid hormones
    C. Sub-acute thyroiditis
    D. Struma ovarii
    E. Trophoblastic disease

47. **A 50-year-old woman presented to clinic with lethargy and weight loss. On examination, she was noticed to have mild tremors and a heart rate of 70 beats/minute.**

    ```
    Investigations:
       free T4   18.5 pmol/L (11.5-19.7)
       free T3   6.2 pmol/L (3.5-6.5)
       TSH       0.05 mU/L (0.35-5.5)
    ```

    A RAIU scan was planned for the following week.

    Which one of the following is the most appropriate management plan for her while she was waiting for a thyroid RAIU scan?

    A. Carbimazole
    B. Lugol's iodine
    C. Observe
    D. Propanolol
    E. Propylthiouracil

48. **A 22-year-old university student presented to the thyroid clinic with symptoms of anxiety, weight loss, menstrual irregularities, and palpitations. She had a strong family history of thyroid dysfunction and autoimmune disease. On examination, she had tremors, tachycardia, bilateral proptosis, and a diffuse enlargement of thyroid gland.**

```
Investigations:
   free T4                  35.5 pmol/L (11.5-19.7)
   free T3                  15.0 pmol/L (3.5-6.5)
   TSH                      <0.01 mU/L (0.35-5.5)
   TSH receptor antibody  positive
```

A diagnosis of Graves' thyrotoxicosis was made and she was started on carbimazole therapy. She was quite keen to know her chances of going into disease remission.

Which one of the following factors is predictive of development of remission in Graves' disease?

A. Age >40 years

B. Anti-TPO antibody titre

C. Lower free T3 levels

D. Male sex

E. Positive family history

49. **A 33-year-old woman, who was 20 weeks pregnant, presented to the antenatal clinic with symptoms of palpitations, increased sweating, and panic episodes. She was diagnosed as having Graves' disease about 3 months ago and required carbimazole 40 mg/day. On examination, she had heart rate of 122 beats/minute, bilateral tremors, and a small goitre.**

```
TFT results:
   free T4  30.6 pmol/L (11.5-19.7)
   free T3  12.8 pmol/L (3.5-6.5)
   TSH      <0.01 mU/L (0.35-5.5)
```

Which one of the following is the most appropriate management approach in her case?

A. Elective surgery

B. Increase carbimazole dose

C. Propanolol

D. RAIA post-delivery

E. Switch to propylthiouracil

50. **A 36-year-old woman presented to the endocrine clinic with features of palpitations and weight loss. She had a background history of Graves' disease, which was treated with carbimazole therapy for 1 year and she had been in disease remission for the last 2 years. On examination, she had tremors, tachycardia, and increased sweating.**

```
TFT results:
  free T4   25.6 pmol/L (11.5-19.7)
  free T3   9.4 pmol/L (3.5-6.5)
  TSH       <0.01 mU/L (0.35-5.5)
```

In view of a relapse of her Graves' disease, she received counselling for RAIA.

Which one of the following is associated with an increase in radio-resistance of thyroid gland prior to RAI therapy?

A. Carbimazole
B. Levothyroxine
C. Lugol's iodine
D. Methimazole
E. Propylthiouracil

51. **A 52-year-old presented to the thyroid clinic with symptoms of anxiety and palpitations. She had a background history of Graves' disease that was treated with a 6-month course of block and replacement therapy, and had been in remission for the last 1 year. On examination, she had tachycardia with a heart rate of 90 beats/minute, bilateral tremors, and a small goitre.**

```
TFT results:
  free T4   22.5 pmol/L (11.5-19.7)
  free T3   8.1 pmol/L (3.5-6.5)
  TSH       0.08 mU/L (0.35-5.5)
```

Which one of the following is the most appropriate definitive management approach in her case?

A. Carbimazole
B. Elective surgery
C. Observe
D. Propanolol
E. RAIA therapy

52. **A 35-year-old woman presented to her GP with symptoms of lethargy, palpitations, and anxiety. She had recently suffered from a flu-like illness that had lasted for about a week. On examination, she had tremors, tachycardia (a heart rate of 110 beats/minute), and increased sweating. There were no eye signs of GO and her systemic examination was unremarkable.**

```
Investigations:
   free T4               21.0 pmol/L (11.5-19.7 pmol/L)
   TSH                   0.15 mU/L (0.35-5.5 mU/L)
   CRP                   90 mg/L (<6 mg/L)
   TSH receptor antibody negative
```

Which one of the following is the most appropriate management approach in her case?

A. Carbimazole

B. Carbimazole and propanolol

C. Propanolol

D. RAIA

E. Subtotal thyroidectomy

53. **A 57-year-old man presented to the thyroid clinic with ongoing symptoms of palpitations, increased sweating, and weight loss. He had a background history of hyperthyroidism, secondary to a multi-nodular goitre, which was treated with RAI therapy about 10 months ago.**

```
TFT results:
   free T4  24.5 pmol/L (11.5-19.7)
   free T3  8.2 pmol/L (3.5-6.5)
   TSH      0.03 mU/L (0.35-5.5)
```

Which one of the following is the most appropriate management approach in his case?

A. Carbimazole

B. Elective thyroidectomy

C. Observe

D. Propanolol

E. RAIA

54. **A 25-year-old woman was incidentally detected to have a thyroid nodule measuring 0.8 cm on an ultrasound of the neck arranged by her GP. She had no previous history of radiation exposure and there was no family history of thyroid-related malignancy. On examination, she had no visible or palpable goitre, or cervical lymph nodes.**

```
TFT results:
  free T4  15.3 pmol/L (11.5–19.7)
  TSH       2.5 mU/L (0.35–5.5)
```

Which one of the following is the most appropriate management approach in her case?

A. Manage in primary care
B. Measure calcitonin
C. Measure thyroglobulin
D. Non-urgent referral for FNAC
E. Urgent referral for FNAC

55. **A 17-year-old boy presented to the thyroid clinic with a painless lump in the neck that he had noticed a few weeks previously. He had a previous history of cranial lymphoma as a child, which was treated with radiotherapy and chemotherapy. On examination, he had a 1.5-cm firm thyroid nodule palpable with no cervical lymphadenopathy. His TFT results were within normal range.**

All of the following are considered to be risk factors for the development of thyroid cancer except?

A. Endemic goitre
B. Familial adenomatous polyposis
C. Family history of thyroid adenoma
D. Hashimoto's thyroiditis
E. Reidel's thyroiditis

56. **A 55-year-old woman was reviewed in the multidisciplinary thyroid cancer clinic with incidentally detected thyroid nodule. On examination, she had a firm 4.5-cm left-sided thyroid nodule together with enlarged cervical lymph nodes. Her TFT results were within the normal range and FNAC results confirmed a follicular carcinoma with vascular invasion.**

All of the following are considered to be poor prognostic markers for differentiated thyroid cancer except?

A. Age >40 years
B. Female gender
C. Poorly-differentiated tumour
D. Tumour size
E. Vascular invasion

57. **A 42-year-old woman was reviewed in the multidisciplinary thyroid cancer clinic with a rapidly enlarging neck swelling and hoarseness of the voice. She had a family history of thyroid dysfunction and adenoma. On examination, she had a 2.5-cm right-sided thyroid nodule with no palpable cervical lymph nodes. Her TFT results were within the normal range and FNAC confirmed the diagnosis of papillary thyroid cancer. She underwent an elective total thyroidectomy followed by a ^{131}I ablation.**

   How soon after total thyroidectomy, Tg levels should be measured?

   A. Immediately after the operation
   B. After 1 week
   C. After 6 weeks
   D. After 6 months
   E. After 1 year

58. **A 25-year-old woman was incidentally detected to have a 0.6-cm thyroid nodule on ultrasound of the neck. FNAC confirmed the diagnosis of a well-differentiated papillary thyroid cancer. Further investigations confirmed the absence of any regional or distant metastasis of the tumour. She subsequently underwent a lobectomy with complete resection of the tumour.**

   Which one of the following is the most appropriate further management approach in her case?

   A. External beam radiotherapy
   B. ^{131}I ablation post-operatively
   C. Measurement of stimulated Tg
   D. PET scan
   E. Whole body scan after 6 months

59. **A 22-year-old woman presented with a rapidly enlarging neck lump. She had a strong family history of thyroid dysfunction and elevated calcium. On examination, she had a 2.5-cm hard thyroid nodule without any palpable cervical lymph nodes. Further investigations showed elevated calcitonin levels and FNAC confirmed the diagnosis of medullary thyroid cancer.**

   Which one the following is the most appropriate step in her further management?

   A. Chemotherapy
   B. External beam radiotherapy
   C. Somatostatin analogues
   D. Total thyroidectomy and lymph node dissection
   E. Total thyroidectomy followed by ^{131}I ablation

60. A 50-year-old woman was reviewed in the thyroid cancer clinic on a routine follow-up visit. She had undergone a total thyroidectomy followed by ^{131}I ablation for a well-differentiated 2.5-cm follicular carcinoma (pT2N0M0), 3 years previously. During this clinic visit, her physical and systemic examination was normal.

```
Investigations:
    free T4          20.9 pmol/L (11.5-19.7)
    TSH              0.04 mU/L (0.35-5.5)
    Tg               detectable
    Tg antibodies    negative
    RAI scan         negative
```

Which one of the following is the most appropriate further management approach in her case?

A. Decrease thyroxine dose

B. Increase thyroxine dose

C. PET scan

D. Switch to liothyronine

E. Ultrasound of the neck

61. A 52-year-old woman presented to the endocrine clinic with symptoms of palpitations, restlessness, diarrhoea, and weight loss. On examination, she had mild tremors in the hands, no eye signs of Graves' eye disease, and no visible/palpable goitre.

```
Investigations:
   free T4                30.5 pmol/L (11.5-19.7)
   TSH                    <0.01 mU/L (0.35-5.5)
   TSH receptor antibody  negative
```

She underwent RAIU scan (see Figure 2.2).

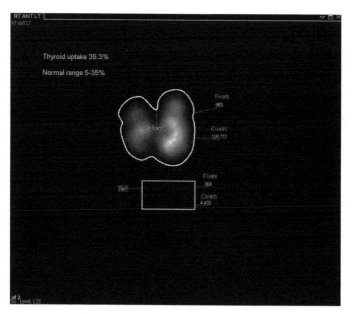

Figure 2.2 Radioactive iodine uptake scan

Which one of the following is the most appropriate management approach in her case based on her clinical profile?

A. Observation

B. Propanolol

C. Propylthiouracil

D. RAIA

E. Thyroidectomy

62. **A 32-year-old woman presented to the clinic with a 4-week history of flu-like symptoms, difficulty in swallowing, and pain in neck region. On examination, she was noticed to have bilateral tremors and tenderness in the neck on palpation. Her heart rate was 84 beats/minute, regular.**

```
Investigations:
  free T4  20.5 pmol/L (11.5-19.7)
  free T3  5.5 pmol/L (3.5-6.5)
  TSH      0.12 mU/L (0.35-5.5)
```

She underwent RAIU scan (^{123}I) (see Figure 2.3).

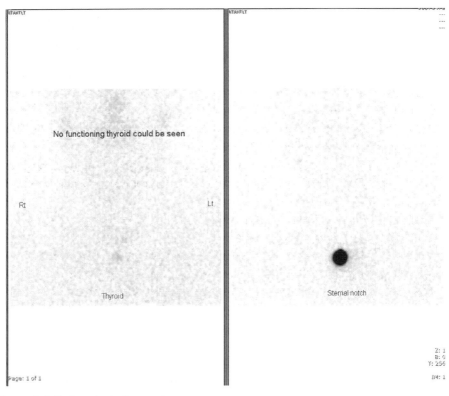

Figure 2.3 Radioactive iodine uptake scan

Reproduced with permission from Dr Nimit Goyal, Consultant Radiologist, Royal Gwent Hospital, Newport, UK

Which one of the following is the most appropriate management plan for her based on her clinical profile?

A. Anti-inflammatory agents

B. Carbimazole

C. Elective thyroidectomy

D. Prednisolone

E. RAIA

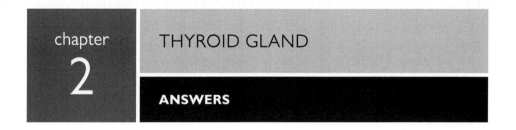

chapter

2

THYROID GLAND

ANSWERS

1. E. The thyroid gland is usually the first endocrine gland to develop in the body at around 24 days of gestation. It originates as proliferation of endodermal epithelium on the floor of the developing pharynx, with some contribution from the lateral pharyngeal pouches. The foetal thyroid gland is connected to the tongue by the thyroglossal duct, which subsequently solidifies and becomes completely obliterated by 8–10 weeks of gestation. During development, the posterior aspect of the thyroid gland becomes associated with the parathyroid gland and the para-follicular cells (C cells) derived from the ultimo-branchial body. The ultimo-branchial body is believed to originate from the fifth pharyngeal pouch, with infiltration of cells migrating from the neural crest.

Jameson JL, De Groot LJ. Endocrinology. Adult and paediatric (6th edn). Saunders Elsevier, 2010.

Kratzsch J. Thyroid gland development and defects. Best Practice and Research in Clinical Endocrinology and Metabolism, 2008; 22: 57–75.

2. E. TBG has a high affinity for thyroid hormones and carries about 70% of circulating T3 and T4. TBG levels are influenced by a wide array of clinical conditions and medications as shown in Table 2.1.

Table 2.1 Clinical conditions and medication that influence TBG levels

TBG increased	TBG decreased
New born	Androgens
Oestrogen	Large-dose steroids, Cushing's disease
Tamoxifen	Chronic liver disease
Hepatitis A, chronic active hepatitis	Severe systemic illness
Biliary cirrhosis	Active acromegaly
Oral contraceptive pills	Nephrotic syndrome
Pregnancy	Drugs: phenytoin

Jameson JL, De Groot LJ. Endocrinology. Adult and paediatric (6th edn). Saunders Elsevier, 2010.

Turner HE, Wass JA. Oxford handbook of endocrinology and diabetes (2nd edn). Oxford University Press, 2009.

3. E. Thyroid hormone resistance syndrome is characterized by elevated FT4 and FT3 in the presence of a non-suppressed TSH. Resistance to thyroid hormone can be:

- Generalized resistance.
- Selective pituitary resistance.
- Selective peripheral resistance

Patients are usually asymptomatic, although there may be a small goitre palpable in patients with selective pituitary resistance. Other clinical features that may be present include short stature, hyperactivity and inattention with or without learning difficulties. Most patients do not require any treatment, although β-blockers can be used to ameliorate symptoms mostly in patients with selective pituitary resistance.

Thyroid hormone resistance can be distinguished from a TSH-secreting adenoma (TSHoma) on the basis of low α subunit to TSH molar ratio of <1, dynamic test using TRH stimulation (an increase of TSH secretion seen in thyroid hormone resistance), and MRI pituitary.

Chatterjee VK. Resistance to thyroid hormones. Hormone Research 1997; 48 (Suppl 4): 43–46.

McDermott MT, Ridgway EC. Thyroid hormone resistance syndromes. American Journal of Medicine 1993; 94: 424–432.

4. C. Thyroid hormones circulate mostly bound to TBG, TBPA, and albumin. It is the free hormones (FT3 and FT4) that are biologically active and transported within the cells (by passive diffusion or specific carriers) to bind to specific receptors in the cell nucleus. The nuclear receptors for the thyroid hormone belong to a family of receptors that are similar to receptors for glucocorticoids, oestrogens, retinoic acid, and mineralocorticoids.

The thyroid hormone receptor is encoded by two genes: TRα and TRβ, located on chromosomes 17 and 4, respectively. These genes further produce two products each (TRα1 and 2; TRβ1 and 2). Mutations in the ligand-binding domain of TRβ are associated with thyroid hormone resistance syndrome. Most of these mutations have an autosomal dominant mode of inheritance.

Chatterjee VK. Resistance to thyroid hormones. Hormone Research 1997; 48 (Suppl 4): 43–46.

McDermott MT, Ridgway EC. Thyroid hormone resistance syndromes. American Journal of Medicine 1993; 94: 424–32.

5. A. TSH is a glycoprotein synthesized and secreted by thyrotrophs of the anterior pituitary gland. It is composed of two subunits, α and β, linked together by non-covalent bonds. α subunit is common between other glycoprotein hormones, such as FSH, LH, and β-hCG, while the β subunit confers it specific biological activity and binding properties. TSH synthesis and release may be stimulated/inhibited by certain hormones and drugs as shown in Table 2.2.

Table 2.2 Predominant effect of various hormones on TSH secretion

TSH stimulation	TSH inhibition
Thyrotropin-releasing hormone	Thyroid hormones and analogues
Opioids	Dopamine agonists
Arginine-vasopressin	Gastrin
Glucagon-like peptide 1	Somatostatin
Leptin	Glucocorticoids
	Growth hormone

Jameson JL and De Groot LJ. Endocrinology. Adult and paediatric (6th edn). Saunders Elsevier, 2010.

Turner HE and Wass JA. Oxford handbook of endocrinology and diabetes (2nd edn). Oxford University Press, 2009.

6. E. TSH binds to the TSH-R, which is a trans-membrane G protein-coupled receptor on the thyroid cells membrane. The binding activates the G protein-linked adenyl cyclase-cAMP signalling cascades. TSH-R also has binding sites for stimulating (TSH-R Ab, stim) and blocking antibodies (TSH-R Ab block), which are seen in patients with Graves' disease and autoimmune atrophic

thyroiditis, respectively. Mutations of TSH-R can lead to either hyperthyroidism (due to spontaneous activation of receptor) or hypothyroidism (due to TSH resistance).

Jameson JL and De Groot LJ. Endocrinology. Adult and paediatric (6th edn). Saunders Elsevier, 2010.

7. D. Thyroglobulin (Tg) is a dimeric glycoprotein that is synthesized and utilized within the thyroid
gland. Tg plays a crucial role in the synthesis of thyroid hormones, which takes place at the interface
between follicle cells and the colloid. Low levels of Tg are seen in thyrotoxicosis factitia in contrast
to high Tg levels and depressed uptake on scintigraphy seen in patients with thyroiditis.

Jameson JL and De Groot LJ. Endocrinology. Adult and paediatric (6th edn). Saunders Elsevier, 2010.

Luo Y, Ishido Y, Hiroi N, et al. The emerging roles of thyroglobulin. Advances in Endocrinology, 2014;
2014: Article ID 189194. Available at: http://dx.doi.org/10.1155/2014/189194.

8. C. Sick euthyroid syndrome (SES) or non-thyroidal illness syndrome (NTIS) is described as a
state of thyroid dysfunction often seen in the context of a severe or life-threatening illness (e.g.
septicaemia, organ failure, and end-stage malignancy) in the absence of a previous hypothalamic-
pituitary-thyroid abnormality. It is characterized by low T3 and T4 levels along with elevated levels
of reverse T3.

- TSH levels may be normal, low, or slightly elevated depending on the severity of the illness.
- Total T4 and T3 levels may be altered by binding protein abnormalities.
- Levels of free T3 may be lowered, followed by the lowering of free T4 depending upon the
  severity of the disease.
- Reverse T3 levels are generally increased due to inhibition of normal Type 1 deiodinase en-
  zyme or reduced clearance of reverse T3.

McIver C, Gorman CA. Euthyroid sick syndrome: an overview. Thyroid 1997; 1: 125–32.

9. D. The conversion of T4 to T3 is mediated by the activity of 5' deiodinase enzymes. Deiodination of the outer ring of T4 results in the formation of biologically active T3, while deiodination of
the inner ring leads to formation of metabolically inert reverse T3. Three different types of 5' deiodinase are known to exist as shown in Table 2.3.

Table 2.3 Various 5' deiodinase enzymes and their clinical significance

Type of 5' deiodinase	Site	Action	Role
Type 1	Liver, muscle, kidneys	Acts on outer as well as inner ring of T4	Increased in hyperthyroidism
Type 2	Neurons	Acts on outer ring of T4 to produce T3	Provides T3 to neurons
Type 3	Placenta	Acts on inner ring of T4 to produce RT3	Protects placenta from excess T3 and T4

Bianco AC, Kim BW. Deiodinases: implications of the local control of thyroid hormone function. Journal of Clinical Investigation, 2006; 116: 2571–2579.

Jameson JL, De Groot LJ. Endocrinology. Adult and paediatric (6th edn). Saunders/Elsevier, 2010.

10. B. See Table 2.4, which shows the influence of various medications on thyroid function.

Table 2.4 Influence of various medications on thyroid function

Mechanism of interference	Medications
Increase TBG	Oestrogen, tamoxifen, heroin, methadone, clofibrate
Decrease TBG	Androgens, anabolic steroids, glucocorticoids
Interfere with thyroid hormone binding	Furosemide, mefanamic acid, salicylates phenytoin, diazepam, sulphonylureas, heparin
Inhibit conversion of T4 to T3	Propylthiouracil, glucocorticoids, propranolol, iodinated contrast agents, amiodarone, clomipramine
Increased hepatic metabolism	Phenobarbital, rifampicin, phenytoin, carbamzepine
Decrease T4 absorption or enhance excretion	Cholestyramine, colestipol aluminium hydroxide, ferrous sulphate, sucralfate, amiodarone
Decreased T3/T4 synthesis and/or secretion	Lithium, thionamides propylthiouracil, carbimazole thiocyanate, perchlorate, amiodarone,
Increased T3/T4 synthesis and/or secretion	Iodide, amiodarone, cytokines
Decreased TSH concentration	GH, somatostatin, opiates, dopamine, bromocriptine

Jameson JL, De Groot LJ. Endocrinology. Adult and paediatric (6th edn). Saunders/Elsevier, 2010.

Turner HE, Wass JA. Oxford handbook of endocrinology and diabetes (2nd edn). Oxford University Press, 2009.

11. B. According to the BTA guidelines (2007), most patients with Thy3 cytology have a follicular lesion/suspected follicular neoplasm (see Table 2.5). These patients should be discussed at the thyroid cancer multidisciplinary team (MDT) meeting, with most of them requiring elective lobectomy (the lobe containing the nodule) and completion thyroidectomy if histology confirms carcinoma.

Table 2.5 Thy classification for thyroid cancer

FNAC result	Interpretation	Action
Thy 1	Non-diagnostic	Repeat FNAC
Thy 2	Non-neoplastic	Repeat in 3–6 months (a single well targeted aspirate does not need to be repeated)
Thy3	Follicular adenoma or carcinoma	Discuss at MDT meeting, most require lobectomy
Thy 4	Suspicious of malignancy	Discuss at MDT meeting, most require surgery
Thy 5	Diagnostic of malignancy	Discuss at MDT meeting, may require surgery, and/or radiotherapy, and/or chemotherapy

Data from *Guidelines for Management of Thyroid Cancer*, Second edition, 2007 by British Thyroid Association / Royal College of Physicians available at http://www.british-thyroid-association.org/Guidelines

British Thyroid Association/Royal College of Physicians. Guidelines for management of thyroid cancer (2nd edn). BTA, 2007. Available at http://www.british-thyroid-association.org/Guidelines.

12. D. A Thy2 result on FNAC is suggestive of a non-neoplastic lesion. Generally two non-neoplastic (Thy2) results, 3–6 months apart, are advisable to exclude malignancy.

British Thyroid Association/Royal College of Physicians. Guidelines for management of thyroid cancer (2nd edn). BTA, 2007. Available at http://www.british-thyroid-association.org/Guidelines.

13. D. This gentleman was on the stable dose of thyroxine and developed clinical and biochemical features of hypothyroidism 6 weeks after starting chemotherapy for tuberculosis. Rifampicin is an inducer of hepatic enzymes and accelerates the metabolism of several drugs. In this clinical scenario, his thyroxine dose needs to be increased due to its interaction with rifampicin.

Dong BJ. How medicines affect thyroid function. Western Journal of Medicine, 2000; 172: 102–106.

Surks MI, Sievert R. Drugs and thyroid function. New England Journal of Medicine, 1995; 333: 1688–1694.

14. C. This woman has sub-clinical hyperthyroidism as evidenced by a normal FT4 with a suppressed TSH level. As she has non-specific symptoms together with a measurable TSH level, with no features of an exogenous thyroid dysfunction; hence, the management approach can be conservative at this stage. The presence of an unmeasurable TSH and/or exogenous thyroid dysfunction is an indication for definitive therapy, with most centres managing such patients with RAI in view of solitary/multi-nodular toxic goitre as the commonest aetiology.

Bahn RS, Burch HB, Cooper DS, et al. Hyperthyroidism and other causes of thyrotoxicosis: management guidelines of the American Thyroid Association and American Association of clinical endocrinologists. Endocrine Practice, 2011; 17(3): 456–520.

15. C. The presence of a heterophile antibody that interferes with the assay needs to be considered, and the test should be repeated from a different laboratory, using a different assay method.

Gurnell MK, Halsall DJ, Chatterjee VK. What should be done when thyroid function tests do not make sense? Clinical Endocrinology, 2011; 74: 673–678.

Tate J, Ward G. Interferences in immunoassays. Clinical Biochemist Reviews 2004; 25: 105–120.

16. C. Heparin leads to an increased release of lipoprotein lipase from the vascular endothelium, producing a rise in the levels of free fatty acid (FFA). High levels of FFA inhibit the binding of thyroid hormones to their plasma-binding proteins, producing a rise in measured quantities of thyroid hormones.

Laji K, Ridha B, John R, et al. Abnormal serum free thyroid hormone levels due to heparin administration. Quarterly Journal of Medicine 2001; 94(9): 471–473.

17. B. The main differential diagnosis for elevated TSH, in the presence of normal or high FT4 and FT3, includes a TSHoma and thyroid hormone resistance.

Diagnostic criteria for TSHoma include:

- High SHBG.
- Increased α subunit/TSH molar ratio.
- Blunted or absent response to TRH stimulation.
- MRI findings.

Kienitz T, Quinkler M, Strasburger CJ, et al. Long-term management in five cases of TSH-secreting pituitary adenomas: a single center study and review of the literature. European Journal of Endocrinology, 2007; 157: 39–46.

18. D. Anti-thyroid peroxidase (anti-TPO) antibodies are specific for the auto-antigen TPO, a 105-kDa glycol-protein that catalyses iodine oxidation and Tg tyrosyl iodination reactions in the thyroid gland (see Table 2.6).

Table 2.6 Anti-TPO antibodies status in various conditions

Clinical state	% Anti-TPO positive
Hashimoto's thyroiditis	90–95%
Graves' disease	70–80%
Normal individuals	10–15%

High serum antibodies are found in active phase chronic autoimmune thyroiditis. Thus, an antibody titre can be used to assess disease activity in patients that have developed such antibodies. The majority of anti-TPO antibodies are produced by thyroid infiltrating lymphocytes, with minor contributions from lymph nodes and the bone marrow.

Mariotti S, Caturegli P, Piccolo P, et al. Anti-thyroid peroxidase autoantibodies in thyroid diseases. Journal of Clinical Endocrinology and Metabolism, 1990; 71(3): 661–669.

19. A. Poor compliance with thyroxine replacement commonly causes anomalous TFTs: owing to their differing half-lives, intermittent hormone ingestion may result in normal or even elevated thyroid hormone levels, but fails to normalize TSH. Even more confusingly in this context, a seemingly appropriate increase in thyroxine dosage to perhaps non-physiological levels can normalize TSH, then raising the possibility of the patient being hormone 'resistant'.

However, distinct from the aforementioned context, it is also recognized that thyroxine replacement in physiological dosage to optimize TSH can be associated with mildly elevated FT4, but normal FT3 levels, with this pattern being ascribed to iodothyronine deiodinase type 2 (DIO2) in mediating TH feedback.

Gurnell MK, Halsall DJ, Chatterjee VK. What should be done when thyroid function tests do not make sense? Clinical Endocrinology, 2011; 74: 673–678.

20. B. *Urine*: The 24-hour excretion of T4 in normal adults range from 4 to 13 µg and from 1.8 to 3.7 µg, depending on whether total or only conjugated T4 is measured. Corresponding normal ranges for T3 are 2.0–4.0 µg and 0.4–1.9 µg. Striking seasonal variations have been shown for the urinary excretion of both the hormones.

Amniotic fluid: The T4 concentration in amniotic fluid averages from 0.5 µg/dL with a range from 0.15 to 1.0 µg/dL, and thus is very low when compared with values in maternal and cord serum. The FT4 concentration is, however, twice as high in amniotic fluid relative to serum.

CSF: The concentrations of both T4 and T3 are approximately 50-fold lower than those of serum, however, the concentration of the free forms is similar to those in the serum.

Milk: The total T4 concentration in human milk is around 0.03–0.5 µg/dL. The total T3 concentration ranges from 10 to 200 ng/dL. Thus, it is unlikely that milk would provide a sufficient quantity of thyroid hormone to alleviate hypothyroidism in infant.

Saliva: Levels of T4 in saliva range from 4.2 to 35 ng/dl and do not correlate with the concentration of FT4 in serum.

Tissues: As the response to thyroid hormones is expressed at the cellular level via nuclear receptors, it is logical to assume that human concentrations in tissues should correlate best with their action. Methods for extraction, recovery, and measurements of iodo-thyronines have been developed, but the data is limited. Preliminary work has shown that hormonal levels in tissues such as the liver, kidney, and muscle, usually correlate with that of the serum.

Jameson JL De Groot LJ. Endocrinology. Adult and paediatric (6th edn). Saunders/Elsevier, 2010.

21. A. Amiodarone therapy is commonly associated with thyroid dysfunction and can result in both amiodarone-induced thyrotoxicosis (AIT), as well as amiodarone-induced hypothyroidism (AIH). There are two types of AIT—Type 1 and 2 as described in Table 2.7.

Table 2.7 Major differences between AIT-Type 1 and AIT-Type 2

	AIT Type 1	**AIT Type 2**
Antibody status	Usually positive	Usually negative
Thyroid dysfunction	May be present	Normal gland
Mechanism	Due to excess iodide	Destructive thyroiditis
Thyroid uptake scan	Increased uptake	Reduced uptake
Management	Carbimazole	Steroids

In clinical practice it may not always be possible to distinguish between these two types of amiodarone-induced thyrotoxicosis and the patient may be managed with combination therapy of steroids and thionamides.

Bogazzi F, Bartolena L, Martino E. Approach to patient with amiodarone induced thyrotoxicosis. Journal of Clinical Endocrinology & Metabolism 2010; 95: 2529–2535.

Tsang W, Houlden RL. Amiodarone induced thyrotoxicosis. Canadian Journal of Cardiology 2009; 25: 421–424.

22. B. Amiodarone therapy is commonly associated with thyroid dysfunction and can induce both AIT, as well as AIH. There are two types of AIT—Types 1 and 2. AIT Type 2 usually occurs on background of a normal thyroid gland and associated with reduced uptake on thyroid uptake scan. The treatment of choice in AIT Type 2 is steroid therapy. Amiodarone is essential for her in view of intractable AF so difficult to be stopped. She should be commenced on steroid therapy. In clinical practice patients may require a combination of steroids, as well as carbimazole therapy for AIT, due to practical difficulties in distinguishing between AIT Types 1 and 2.

Bogazzi F, Bartolena L, Martino E. Approach to patient with amiodarone induced thyrotoxicosis. Journal of Clinical Endocrinology & Metabolism 2010; 95: 2529–2535.

Tsang W, Houlden RL. Amiodarone induced thyrotoxicosis. Canadian Journal of Cardiology 2009; 25: 421–4.

23. E. The patient is likely to have Graves' thyrotoxicosis as suggested by features of hyperthyroidism and associated strong family history of autoimmune thyroid disease. Although hyperemesis gravidarum is an important differential diagnosis and presents with similar symptoms, a palpable goitre and audible bruit, on examination is more in favour of a diagnosis of Graves' disease. Her TSH receptor antibody status should be checked and, if positive, she should be commenced on a low dose of carbimazole therapy.

Bahn RS, Burch HB, Cooper DS, et al. Hyperthyroidism and other causes of thyrotoxicosis: management guidelines of the American Thyroid Association and American Association of clinical endocrinologists. Endocrine Practice, 2011; 17(3): 456–520.

Cooper DS, Laurberg P. Hyperthyroidism in pregnancy. Lancet Diabetes Endocrinology 2013; 1(3): 238–249.

Krentz AJ, Redman H, Taylor KG. Hyperthyroidism associated with hyper emesis gravid arum. British Journal of Clinical Practice, 1994; 48(2): 75–76.

24. A. The patient is likely to have Graves' thyrotoxicosis, as suggested by features of hyperthy-roidism and an associated strong family history of autoimmune thyroid disease. Although hyperem-esis gravidarum is an important differential diagnosis and presents with similar symptoms, a palpable goitre and audible bruit on examination is more in favour of diagnosis of Graves' disease. Her TSH receptor antibody status should be checked and, if positive, she should be commenced on a low dose of carbimazole therapy. Carbimazole crosses the placenta and its use is associated with an unproven risk of developing aplasia cutis, oesophageal atresia, and choanal atresia during the first early stages of the first trimester. As a result, some experts avoid using it in women who are of child-bearing age group, although low-dose carbimazole can be used safely from the second trimes-ter onwards and not linked with any foetal thyroid dysfunction.

Cooper DS and Laurberg P. Hyperthyroidism in pregnancy. Lancet Diabetes Endocrinology 2013; 1(3): 238–249.

De Groot L, Abalovich M, Alexander EK, et al. Management of thyroid dysfunction during pregnancy and postpartum: the Endocrine Society guidelines. Journal of Clinical Endocrinology & Metabolism, 2012; 97: 2543–2565.

25. C. This pregnant woman has an elevated TSH, despite being on thyroxine therapy while she is in her first trimester of pregnancy. According to the Endocrine Society guidelines, overt as well as sub-clinical hypothyroidism (TSH >10 mU/L in the presence of normal FT4) is associated with ad-verse foetal and maternal outcomes, and needs to be treated with thyroxine therapy to bring TSH values back to a trimester specific range.

De Groot L, Abalovich M, Alexander EK, et al. Management of thyroid dysfunction during pregnancy and postpartum: the Endocrine Society guidelines. Journal of Clinical Endocrinology & Metabolism, 2012; 97: 2543–2565.

26. B. Graves' disease and hyperemesis gravidarum remain relatively common aetiologies lead-ing to features of nausea, vomiting, and palpitations during the first trimester of pregnancy. TSH receptor antibodies (TRAB) measurement is helpful to distinguish between these two conditions. TRAB should be measured by 22 weeks of gestation and repeated again in third trimester. If levels are elevated 2–3-fold, serial foetal thyroid screening should be done with regular ultrasound at 4–6-week intervals.

De Groot L, Abalovich M, Alexander EK, et al. Management of thyroid dysfunction during pregnancy and postpartum: the Endocrine Society guidelines. Journal of Clinical Endocrinology & Metabolism, 2012; 97: 2543–2565.

27. B. Hyperemesis gravidarum remains an important differential diagnosis for thyroid dysfunction in the first trimester of pregnancy. TRAB should be measured in all patients to distinguish it from Graves' disease. The hyperthyroidism seen in hyperemesis gravidarum is usually transient and anti-thyroid treatment is only required in severely symptomatic patients.

Krentz AJ, Redman H, Taylor KG. Hyperthyroidism associated with hyper emesis gravid arum. British Journal of Clinical Practice 1994; 48(2): 75–76.

28. B. This patient is in the thyrotoxic phase of post-partum thyroiditis (PPT) based on her clinical profile. It is usually characterized by women in the post-partum period presenting with features of thyrotoxicosis lasting for 1–3 months followed by a phase of hypothyroidism, which may last for a period of 6–12 months. It is not uncommon for patients to manifest with only one phase (hyper- or hypothyroidism). It is believed to be mediated by an auto-immune-induced process and is more commonly seen in women with a previous history of auto-immune disease/positive anti-TPO anti-body status or history of previous thyroid dysfunction.

Anti-TPO antibody positivity is the most useful marker for the prediction of post-partum thyroid dysfunction. Symptoms during the thyrotoxic phase of PPT tend to be milder than during hyper-thyroidism due to GD. β-blockers are useful agents for symptom control during the thyrotoxic phase. Asymptomatic women who are not planning a subsequent pregnancy and whose TSH level is between 4 and 10 mIU/L, do not necessarily require intervention and should have their TFTs re-evaluated in 4–8 weeks. When a TSH above the reference range continues post-partum, women should be treated with thyroxine. Women with a TSH between 4 and 10 mIU/L who are either symptomatic or trying to conceive should be treated with thyroxine.

Sakaihara M, Yamada H, Kato EH, et al. Postpartum thyroid dysfunction in women with normal thyroid function during pregnancy. Clinical Endocrinology 2000; 53(4): 487–492.

Stagnaro Green A. Postpartum thyroiditis. Best Practice Research in Clinical Endocrinology & Metabolism, 2004; 18(2): 302–316.

29. B. The following are considered to be risk factors for developing post-partum thyroiditis:

- History of previous post-partum thyroiditis
- Presence of auto-immune disease
- Positive anti-TPO antibody status
- History of previous thyroid dysfunction
- Family history of thyroid disease

De Groot L, Abalovich M, Alexander EK, et al. Management of thyroid dysfunction during pregnancy and postpartum: the Endocrine Society guidelines. Journal of Clinical Endocrinology & Metabolism, 2012; 97: 2543–2565.

30. E. There is no consensus of opinion on routine screening of newly-pregnant women. The focus for screening should be on the following high risk groups:

- Age >30 years
- A family history of autoimmune thyroid disease
- The presence of goitre
- Positive thyroid antibodies status
- The presence of autoimmune disorders
- Infertility
- A history of miscarriage and preterm delivery
- Previous therapeutic head or neck irradiation
- Residence in an iodine deficiency areas

De Groot L, Abalovich M, Alexander EK, et al. Management of thyroid dysfunction during pregnancy and postpartum: the Endocrine Society guidelines. Journal of Clinical Endocrinology & Metabolism, 2012; 97: 2543–2565.

31. C. Based on the symptoms and the signs GO is the most likely aetiology. Patients with GO may be hyper- or euthyroid at presentation. It may present initially with unilateral eye involvement. Orbital cellulitis may present with similar symptoms, although patients may have marked features of sepsis. A carotid-cavernous fistula is characterized by the presence of cranial bruit and dilated episcleral vessels.

Bahn RS. Graves' opthalmopathy. New England Journal of Medicine 2010; 362: 726–738.

Bartalena L, Bardeschi L, Dickinson A, et al. Consensus statement of the European Group on Graves' Orbitopathy (EUGOGO) on management of GO. European Journal of Endocrinology, 2008; 158(3): 273–285.

32. E. Patients with GO with on-going visual symptoms or signs suggestive of active eye disease should have visual acuity and colour vision assessment. A slit lamp examination, fundoscopy, and objective measurement of proptosis may be helpful. The presence of peri-orbital swelling, eyelid erythema, conjunctival redness, chemosis, and restrictions in eye movements are suggestive of active eye disease. The complications of GO include corneal ulceration, optic nerve compression, strabismus (due to medial and inferior rectus muscle involvement) and 4th nerve pseudo-palsy. In the presence of normal visual acuity measurement of visual-evoked potential is not indicated.

Bartalena L, Bardeschi L, Dickinson A, et al. Consensus statement of the European Group on Graves' Orbitopathy (EUGOGO) on management of GO. European Journal of Endocrinology, 2008; 158(3): 273–85.

33. B. The following measures are helpful in the management of mild GO:

- Smoking cessation.
- Use of lubricants such as artificial tears.
- Night-time eyelid taping to prevent exposure keratitis.
- Elevation of head-end of bed to reduce lid swelling.
- Use of prisms for double vision.
- Rarely, botulinum toxin injection.

Soeters MR, Van Zeijl CJ, Boelen A, et al. Optimal management of Graves' orbitopathy: a multidisciplinary approach. Netherlands Journal of Medicine, 2011; 69(7): 302–8.

34. A. The parameters used to determine the CAS score include:

- Active lid swelling (moderate or severe).
- Eyelid erythema.
- Definite conjunctival redness.
- Chemosis.
- Spontaneous orbital pain.
- Gaze-evoked orbital pain.

Bartalena L, Bardeschi L, Dickinson A, et al. Consensus statement of the European Group on Graves' Orbitopathy (EUGOGO) on management of GO. European Journal of Endocrinology, 2008; 158(3): 273–285.

Mourits MP, Prummel MF, Wiersinga WM, et al. Clinical activity score as a guide in the management of patients with Graves' opthalmopathy. Clinical Endocrinology, 1997; 47: 9–14.

35. D. This lady had evidence of moderate–severe GO, based on her symptoms and signs. She needed an urgent referral to the ophthalmologist for further assessment. Her hyperthyroid state needed to be controlled with thionamide therapy together with initiation of systemic steroids. Thyroidectomy is not associated with an improved thyroid eye disease outcome. Radioiodine ablation can be used in the presence of active GO, albeit under cover of steroids. Orbital decompression may be required for severe and sight-threatening GO.

Bartalena L, Marcocci C, Bogazzi F, et al. Use of corticosteroids to prevent progression of Graves' ophthalmopathy after radioiodine therapy for hyperthyroidism. New England Journal of Medicine, 1989; 321(20): 1349–1352.

Bothun ED1, Scheurer RA, Harrison AR, et al. Update on thyroid eye disease and management. Clinical Ophthalmology, 2009; 3: 543–551.

36. C. Patients with severe sight-threatening GO (also known as dysthyroid optic neuropathy) should initially be treated with intravenous glucocorticoids (GCs). If the patients are intolerant to the GCs or fail to respond to these agents, surgical decompression of the orbit is the procedure of choice to alleviate the pressure on the optic nerve.

Bartalena L, Bardeschi L, Dickinson A, et al. Consensus statement of the European Group on Graves' Orbitopathy (EUGOGO) on management of GO. European Journal of Endocrinology, 2008; 158(3): 273–285.

Fichter N, Guthoff RF, Schittkowski MP. Orbital decompression in thyroid eye disease. International Scholarly Research Network: Ophthalmology, 2012; 2012:Article ID 739236. Available at: http://dx.doi.org/10.5402/2012/739236.

37. A. Patients with mild GO may present with eyelid retraction, lid lag (Von Graefe's sign), a widened palpebral fissure during fixation (Dalrymple's sign), and an inability to close the eyelids completely (lagophthalmos). Due to the proptosis, eyelid retraction, and lagophthalmos, the cornea is prone to dryness. The patients may also develop chemosis, epithelial erosions, and kerato-conjunctivitis.

In moderate GO, the signs and symptoms are persistent and increase with the involvement of the intrinsic eye muscles. The inferior rectus muscle is most commonly affected and the patient may experience vertical diplopia on up-gaze and limitation of elevation of the eyes due to fibrosis of the muscle. The medial rectus is the second most-commonly-affected muscle, but multiple muscles may be affected, in an asymmetric fashion.

In severe GO, mass effects and cicatricial changes may occur within the orbit, which may manifest as progressive exophthalmos, restrictive myopathy, and an optic neuropathy. With enlargement of the extra ocular muscle at the orbital apex, the optic nerve is at risk of compression. It can potentially result in a loss of visual acuity, visual field defect, afferent pupillary defect, and loss of colour vision. This is an emergency and requires systemic steroid therapy, and consideration for urgent orbital decompression.

Bahn RS. Graves' opthalmopathy. New England Journal of Medicine 2010; 362: 726–38.

Bothun ED, Scheurer RA, Harrison AR. Update on thyroid eye disease and management. Clinical Opthalmology 2009; 3: 543–51.

38. A. The typical histology of muscle involved in GO involves infiltration of the orbital connective tissue with lymphocytes, plasmocytes, and mastocytes. There is increased release of interleukins, cytokines, and tumour necrosis factor. Orbital fibroblasts are stimulated, resulting in the increased synthesis of mucopolysaccharides, which leads to oedema in extra-ocular muscles. There is also an induction of the lipogenesis by fibroblasts and pre-adipocytes, which can cause an increase in orbital volume and compression due to adipose tissue deposition. Patients with isolated eye involvement due to Graves' disease may be negative to TRAB at the time of initial diagnosis.

Bahn RS, Heufelder AE. Pathogenesis of Graves' opthalmopathy. New England Journal of Medicine, 1993; 329(20): 1468–1475.

39. E. Patients with mild GO may present with eyelid retraction, which is usually the earliest and most common sign. There may be lid lag (Von Graefe's sign), a widened palpebral fissure during fixation (Dalrymple's sign), and an inability to close the eyelids completely (lagophthalmos). Due to the proptosis, eyelid retraction, and lagophthalmos, the cornea is prone to dryness. Patients may also develop chemosis, epithelial erosions, and kerato-conjunctivitis.

Bahn RS. Graves' opthalmopathy. New England Journal of Medicine, 2010; 362(8): 726–738.

40. E. Declining visual acuity is an urgent indication for referral to an ophthalmologist. A formal assessment of visual acuity and colour vision is mandatory in these circumstances.

When to refer to the Ophthalmologists
- Unusual presentations of Graves' eye disease to confirm the diagnosis, e.g. unilateral symptoms and signs, euthyroid eye disease; to be seen within 1–2 months.
- Urgent (to be seen within 1–2 weeks).
  Symptoms:
  - Unexplained drop in vision.
  - Awareness of change in intensity or quality of colour vision in one or both eyes.
  - History of one or both eyes popping out (globe subluxation).
    Signs:
  - Obvious corneal opacity.
  - Cornea still visible when the eyelids are closed.
  - Optic disc swelling.
- Non-urgent (within 1–2 months).
  Symptoms:
  - Eyes abnormally sensitive to light—troublesome or deteriorating over the past 1–2 months.
  - Eyes excessively gritty and not improving after 1 week of topical lubricants.
  - Pain in or behind the eyes: troublesome or deteriorating over the past 1–2 months.
  - Progressive change in appearance of the eyes or eyelids over the past 1–2 months.
  - Appearance of the eyes has changed causing concern to the patient.
  - Seeing two separate images when there should only be one.
  Signs:
  - Troublesome eyelid retraction.
  - Abnormal swelling and/or redness of the eyelids or conjunctiva.
  - Restriction of eye movements or manifest strabismus.
  - Tilting head to avoid double vision.
- No referral is needed for GD with minimal eye symptoms or signs.

NHS Lothian. RefHelp. Lothian referral guideline. Available at: http://www.refhelp.scot.nhs.uk

41. D. The systematic review by Thornton et al. (2007) provided strong evidence for a causal association between smoking and the development of thyroid eye disease. Current-smokers were also more likely to experience disease progression or poorer outcome of treatment.

Thornton J, Kelly SP, Harrison RA, et al. Cigarette smoking and thyroid eye disease: a systematic review. Eye (London), 2007; 21(9): 1135–1145.

42. C. Men undergoing RAI therapy are advised to avoid fathering a child for 3–4 months to allow for turnover of sperm production. On attaining a euthyroid state in both genders, there is no evidence of reduced fertility and/or risk of development of congenital anomalies in offspring.

Bahn RS, Burch HB, Cooper DS, et al. Hyperthyroidism and other causes of thyrotoxicosis: management guidelines of the American Thyroid Association and American Association of Clinical Endocrinologists. Endocrine Practice, 2011; 17(3): 456–520.

43. D. Women undergoing RAIA therapy are advised to delay conception for 4–6 months to allow time to attain a euthyroid status. On attaining a euthyroid state in both genders, there is no evidence of reduced fertility and/or risk of development of congenital anomalies in offspring.

Bahn RS, Burch HB, Cooper DS, et al. Hyperthyroidism and other causes of thyrotoxicosis: management guidelines of the American Thyroid Association and American Association of Clinical Endocrinologists. Endocrine Practice, 2011; 17(3): 456–520.

44. E. The effect of RAIA therapy could take from 6 weeks to 6 months to fully manifest. Treatment failure should only be considered after 6 months have elapsed post-RAI therapy. Patients may need treatment with titrating dose of carbimazole +/− β-blockers after RAI if they become overtly thyrotoxic. A second dose of RAI should be considered only after 6 months following the initial treatment.

Royal College of Physicians. Royal College of Physicians guidelines: radio-iodine in the management of benign thyroid disease. RCP, 2007; 1–41. Available at: http://www.rcplondon.ac.uk/sites/default/files/documents/radioiodine-management-benign-thyroid-disease.pdf

45. E. RAI has been used successfully for the treatment of thyrotoxicosis for more than 50 years. Patients who have received this treatment have been studied very carefully. There is no increased risk of developing cancer as a result of this treatment.

Franklyn JA, Masionneuve P, Sheppard M, et al. Cancer incidence and mortality after radio-iodine treatment for hyperthyroidism: population based cohort study. Lancet, 1990; 353(9170): 2111–2115.

46. E. Thyrotoxicosis can be associated with:
- Normal/increased uptake on RAIU scan:
  - Graves' disease.
  - Toxic nodular or multinodular goitre.
  - Trophoblastic disease.
  - TSH-producing pituitary adenomas.
  - Resistance to thyroid hormone (T3 receptor mutation).
- Near-absent uptake on RAIU scan:
  - Painless (silent) thyroiditis/acute thyroiditis.
  - AIT Type 2.
  - Subacute (granulomatous, de Quervain's) thyroiditis.
  - Iatrogenic thyrotoxicosis.
  - Factitious ingestion of thyroid hormone.
  - Struma ovarii.

Bahn RS, Burch HB, Cooper DS, et al. Hyperthyroidism and other causes of thyrotoxicosis: management guidelines of the American Thyroid Association and American Association of Clinical Endocrinologists. Endocrine Practice, 2011; 17(3): 456–520.

Kim M, Ladenson P. Thyroid. In: Goldman L, Schafer AI (eds), Cecil Medicine (24th edn). Saunders Elsevier, 2011; chapter 233.

Salvatore D, Davies TF, Schlumberger MJ, et al. Thyroid physiology and diagnostic evaluation of patients with thyroid disorders. In: Melmed S, Polonsky KS, Larsen PR, et al. (eds), *Williams Textbook of Endocrinology* (12th edn). Saunders Elsevier, 2011; chapter 11.

47. C. Carbimazole therapy should be stopped/or not commenced (whenever it is possible) before a RAIU scan to allow TSH to recover, resulting in better uptake of iodine. RAIU is indicated when the diagnosis is in question (except during pregnancy) and helps to distinguish various aetiologies of thyrotoxicosis having elevated or normal uptake over the thyroid gland from the ones that display a reduced or near-absent uptake.

- RAIU is usually elevated in patients with GD, and normal or high in toxic nodular goitre. The pattern of RAIU in GD is diffuse unless there are coexistent nodules or fibrosis.

- The pattern of uptake in a patient with a single toxic nodule generally shows focal uptake in the adenoma with suppressed uptake in the surrounding areas and contra-lateral thyroid tissue.
- RAIU in multi-nodular goitre demonstrates multiple areas of focal increased and suppressed uptake.
- RAIU will be near zero in patients with painless, post-partum, or sub-acute thyroiditis, factitious ingestion of thyroid hormone, and recent excess iodine intake.
- RAIU may be low after exposure to iodinated contrast in the preceding 1–2 months or with ingestion of a diet unusually rich in iodine, such as seaweed soup or kelp.
- When exposure to excess iodine is suspected (e.g. when the RAIU is lower than expected), but not well established from the history, assessment of urinary iodine concentration may be helpful.

Bahn RS, Burch HB, Cooper DS, et al. Hyperthyroidism and other causes of thyrotoxicosis: management guidelines of the American Thyroid Association and American Association of Clinical Endocrinologists. Endocrine Practice, 2011; 17(3): 456–520.

Kim M, Ladenson P. Thyroid. In: Goldman L, Schafer AI (eds), Cecil Medicine (24th edn). Saunders Elsevier, 2011; chapter 233.

Salvatore D, Davies TF, Schlumberger MJ, et al. Thyroid physiology and diagnostic evaluation of patients with thyroid disorders. In: Melmed S, Polonsky KS, Larsen PR, et al. (eds), *Williams Textbook of Endocrinology* (12th edn). Saunders Elsevier, 2011; chapter 11.

48. C. The principal factors that predict remission in GD include:

- Female sex.
- Size of goitre.
- Serum FT3 and TSH levels.
- Titre of TSH receptor antibodies.
- Age at diagnosis: less chances of remission if age>40 years at diagnosis.

Vitti P, Rago T, Chiovato L, et al. Clinical features of patients with Graves' disease undergoing remission after antithyroid drug treatment. Thyroid, 1997; 7(3): 369–375.

Young ET, Steel NR, Taylor JJ, et al. Prediction of remission after anti-thyroid drug treatment in Graves' disease. Quarterly Journal of Medicine, 1988; 66(250): 175–189.

49. A. Subtotal thyroidectomy may be indicated during pregnancy as a therapy for maternal GD if:

- Patients develop severe adverse reaction to anti-thyroid drug therapy.
- Persistently high doses of anti-thyroid drugs are required (over 30 mg/day of carbimazole or 450 mg/day of propylthiouracil).
- Patients who are non-adherent to anti-thyroid drug therapy and have uncontrolled hyperthyroidism.

The optimal timing of surgery is in the second trimester.

De Groot L, Abalovich M, Alexander EK, et al. Management of thyroid dysfunction during pregnancy and postpartum: an Endocrine Society clinical practice guideline. Journal of Clinical Endocrinology & Metabolism, 2012; 97: 2543–2565.

50. E. Propylthiouracil (PTU) treatment has been linked with radio-resistant effect, resulting in RAI treatment failure. It is believed that the radio-resistance associated with PTU is due to the presence of a sulphydryl group, which is not present in methimazole and carbimazole. Treatment failure rates are higher in patients whose last PTU dose is within 1 week prior to ^{131}I therapy. The duration of PTU therapy has also been linked with higher chances of RAI failure.

Yau JS, Chu KS, Li JK, et al. Usage of a fixed dose of radioactive iodine for the treatment of hyperthyroidism: one-year outcome in a regional hospital in Hong Kong. Hong Kong Medical Journal, 2009; 15: 267–273.

51. B. RAIA therapy is the treatment of choice for patients with a relapse of GD in the absence of contraindications, such as pregnancy and active severe GO.

Bahn RS, Burch HB, Cooper DS, et al. Hyperthyroidism and other causes of thyrotoxicosis: management guidelines of the American Thyroid Association and American Association of Clinical Endocrinologists. Endocrine Practice, 2011; 17(3): 456–520.

52. C. This woman has presented with features of a viral thyroiditis as evidenced by recent flu-like illness, symptoms and signs of hyperthyroidism, and raised inflammatory markers. The hyperthyroidism seen in patients with viral thyroiditis is usually transient and self-remitting. β-blockers are generally used for the symptom control, thionamide therapy is usually not required unless there are moderate-severe clinical features of hyperthyroidism.

Bahn RS, Burch HB, Cooper DS, et al. Hyperthyroidism and other causes of thyrotoxicosis: management guidelines of the American Thyroid Association and American Association of Clinical Endocrinologists. Endocrine Practice, 2011; 17(3): 456–520.

[In particular the section on sub-acute thyroiditis.]

53. E. If hyperthyroidism persists beyond 6 months following ^{131}I therapy for toxic multinodular goitre or toxic adenoma, retreatment with RAI is suggested. A few patients who have features of mild–moderate hyperthyroidism post-RAIA therapy may require carbimazole therapy until the RAI is effective. Surgery may be required in severe or refractory cases of persistent hyperthyroidism due to toxic multinodular goitre or adenoma.

Bahn RS, Burch HB, Cooper DS, et al. Hyperthyroidism and other causes of thyrotoxicosis: management guidelines of the American Thyroid Association and American Association of Clinical Endocrinologists. Endocrine Practice, 2011; 17(3): 456–520.

Royal College of Physicians. Royal College of Physicians guidelines: radio-iodine in the management of benign thyroid disease. RCP, 2007; 1–41. Available at: http://www.rcplondon.ac.uk/sites/default/files/documents/radioiodine-management-benign-thyroid-disease.pdf

54. A. Thyroid nodules are mostly benign and may be detected by palpation in 2% of men and 10% of women, while small nodules may be detected by ultrasonography of neck in up to 60% of the population (see Table 2.8).

Table 2.8 Referral criteria for management of thyroid lumps/nodules

Manage in primary care	Non-urgent referral	Urgent referral	Same day referral
Thyroid lump or goitre, which remains unchanged in size (with no risk factors for cancer)	Abnormal TFT	Unexplained hoarseness of voice and/or presence of cervical lymph nodes	Presence of stridor
Non-palpable thyroid nodules <1cm (incidentally detected)	Sudden onset of pain in thyroid lump	Thyroid nodule in a child	
	Gradually enlarging (over months)	Rapidly enlarging (over weeks) painless thyroid mass	

British Thyroid Association and Royal College of Physicians. Guidelines for the management of thyroid cancer (2nd edn). BTA/RCP, 2007. Available at: http://www.british-thyroid-association.org

55. E. According to the guidelines issued by British Thyroid Association on the management of thyroid cancer, the following are considered to be risk factors for thyroid cancer:

- History of neck irradiation in childhood.
- Endemic goitre.
- Hashimoto's thyroiditis (risk of lymphoma).
- Family or personal history of thyroid adenoma.
- Cowden's syndrome.
- Familial adenomatous polyposis.
- Familial thyroid cancer.

A thyroid nodule is more likely to be malignant if it is associated with any of the following features:

- Age <10 years or >40 years.
- A firm, solitary, non-toxic nodule.
- Hoarseness of voice.
- Palpable cervical lymph node.
- Micro-calcification on ultrasonography.

British Thyroid Association and Royal College of Physicians. Guidelines for the management of thyroid cancer (2nd edn). BTA/RCP, 2007. Available at: http://www.british-thyroid-association.org

56. B. The following factors are linked with poor prognosis in a differentiated thyroid cancer:

- Age <10 years or >40 years.
- Male gender.
- Cellular differentiation and vascular invasion on histology.
- Tumour size.
- Tumour extent (lymph node involvement/metastasis).

British Thyroid Association and Royal College of Physicians. Guidelines for the management of thyroid cancer (2nd edn). BTA/RCP, 2007. Available at: http://www.british-thyroid-association.org

57. C. The majority of patients with papillary thyroid cancer >1 cm in diameter or with a high risk of follicular thyroid cancer should undergo a total or near-total thyroidectomy.

- Serum Tg levels should be checked at least 6 weeks after surgery to avoid a false positive test results.
- An elective ^{131}I ablation should be arranged within 3–6 weeks of thyroidectomy.
- Suppressive dose of thyroxine should be started (3 days after ^{131}I ablation) with the aim of keeping TSH levels <0.1 mIU/L.
- A whole-body scan and stimulated Tg measurement should be arranged after stopping thyroxine for at least 4 weeks after 6 months of ^{131}I ablation.

British Thyroid Association and Royal College of Physicians. Guidelines for the management of thyroid cancer (2nd edn). BTA/RCP, 2007. Available at: http://www.british-thyroid-association.org

58. C. —Measurement of stimulated Tg

- Patients with low-risk follicular cancer or papillary cancer ≤ 1 cm may be treated with thyroid lobectomy.
- ^{131}I ablation post-operatively is not needed.
- Suppressive dose of thyroxine should be started with the aim to keep TSH levels <0.5 mIU/L.
- Tg measurement after TSH stimulation should be arranged at least 6 months after thyroidectomy.
- A whole body scan is usually not required.

British Thyroid Association and Royal College of Physicians. Guidelines for the management of thyroid cancer (2nd edn). BTA/RCP, 2007. Available at: http://www.british-thyroid-association.org

59. D. According to the British Thyroid Association (BTA) guidelines regarding management of medullary thyroid cancer (MTC):

- The initial evaluation of suspected MTC patients should include FNAC and plasma calcitonin measurement.
- The patient should be offered genetic counselling and *RET* gene mutation analysis
- Screen for MEN 2A and 2B.
- Screen for phaeochromocytomas and primary hyperparathyroidism.
- Arrange for total thyroidectomy and level 6 lymph node dissection.
- Prophylactic surgery should be considered in disease-free carriers of germ line *RET* mutation. Surgery should be performed before the age of 5 years for MEN 2A patients and by the age of 1 year in MEN 2B patients.
- Lifelong follow-up with monitoring of calcitonin levels.

British Thyroid Association and Royal College of Physicians. Guidelines for the management of thyroid cancer (2nd edn). BTA/RCP, 2007. Available at: http://www.british-thyroid-association.org

60. E. Tg is secreted by normal, as well as cancerous thyroid cells. Detectable Tg results may be seen in patients with thyroid remnant, residual or recurrent tumour, or in presence of endogenous Tg antibodies

The following points sum up the British Thyroid Association (BTA) guidelines for Tg measurement in patients with differentiated thyroid cancer.

- To ensure continuity in monitoring, clinicians should use the same laboratory and Tg assay on a long-term basis.
- Tg Ab should be measured simultaneously with serum Tg.
- There is normally no need to measure serum Tg more frequently than 3-monthly during routine follow-up.
- For patients in remission measure Tg and TSH on annual basis.
- There is no need for TSH stimulation if the basal serum Tg is already detectable.
- Patients in whom the basal Tg remains persistently detectable (while on suppressive levothyroxine therapy) or rises with subsequent assessments, require further evaluation.
- In the presence of a rising Tg and rising Tg levels there are three potential approaches:
  - No action until the patient is symptomatic.
  - Empirical use of ^{131}I therapy.
  - Investigations to localize disease recurrence which include neck ultrasound, CT scan of lungs (if neck ultrasound is normal), ^{99m}Tc bone scan (if neck ultrasound, as well as CT lungs normal) in that order. A PET scan may be used if all the previously mentioned investigations are normal.

British Thyroid Association and Royal College of Physicians. Guidelines for the management of thyroid cancer (2nd edn). BTA/RCP, 2007. Available at: http://www.british-thyroid-association.org

61. D. This woman has clinical and biochemical features of hyperthyroidism with increased uptake on thyroid uptake scan, consistent with a diagnosis of toxic nodular goitre. RAIA therapy is the treatment of choice in this clinical scenario.

Bahn RS, Burch HB, Cooper DS, et al. Hyperthyroidism and other causes of thyrotoxicosis: management guidelines of the American Thyroid Association and American Association of Clinical Endocrinologists. Endocrine Practice, 2011; 17(3): 456–520.

62. A. The clinical profile of flu-like symptoms, neck pain, mild features of hyperthyroidism, and lack of uptake on RAIU scan is consistent with a diagnosis of subacute/de Quervains thyroiditis. It is usually a self-limiting disease and may show triphasic clinical course (hyperthyroidism, hypothyroidism followed by euthyroid state). The hyperthyroid state is believed to be due to destruction of thyroid follicles (due to inflammatory process) resulting in the release of preformed thyroid hormones into the circulation. Patients may need β-blockers, such as propanolol for symptom relief and anti-inflammatory agents. This stage may last for 6–8 weeks and is usually followed by hypothyroid or euthyroid state. Anti-thyroid medications are usually not required, as 90–95% of patients show complete recovery of thyroid function.

Bahn RS, Burch HB, Cooper DS, et al. Hyperthyroidism and other causes of thyrotoxicosis: management guidelines of the American Thyroid Association and American Association of Clinical Endocrinologists. Endocrine Practice, 2011; 17(3): 456–520.

1. **The four parathyroid glands play a key role in calcium homeostasis by secreting parathyroid hormone (PTH).**

   Which one of the following statement regarding parathyroid gland/PTH physiology is correct?

   A. 1, 25-dihydoxy vitamin D is the main storage form of vitamin D
   B. Parathyroid glands develop from 5th and 6th pharyngeal pouches
   C. PTH enhances the reabsorption of calcium in the proximal renal tubule
   D. PTH reduces the absorption of calcium from the bones
   E. PTH reduces the reabsorption of phosphate in the proximal renal tubule

2. **A 26-year-old care home worker was referred to the combined Endocrinology–Obstetric antenatal clinic by her GP due to incidental finding of low calcium in her routine blood tests while she was 32 weeks pregnant. There was no significant past medical history and she was not on any regular medication.**

   ```
   Investigations:
      total calcium   2.10 mmol/L (2.2–2.6)
      phosphate       0.92 mmol/L (0.8–1.5)
      PTH             2.6 pmol/L (1.6–7.2)
      total protein   54 g/L (65–75)
      albumin         28 g/L (35–40)
   ```

   Which one of the following statements regarding calcium homeostasis during pregnancy is incorrect?

   A. About 25–30 g of calcium is provided by the mother to support foetal skeletal development
   B. Calcium is actively transported across the placenta, facilitated by PTH-related protein (PTHrP)
   C. Free ionized calcium levels increase in pregnancy
   D. The placenta produces 1,25 dihydroxy vitamin D, which results in increased intestinal calcium absorption
   E. Total calcium concentration falls in pregnancy due to physiological hypoalbuminaemia

3. **A 65-year-old retired nurse was referred to the endocrine clinic by her primary care physician in view of incidentally-detected hypercalcaemia. She had no significant past medical history and was not taking any regular medications. Her general physical and systemic examination was unremarkable.**

    ```
    Investigations:
      Urea                   7.5 mg/dL (5-9)
      Creatinine             98 µmol/L (60-115)
      Calcium                2.8 mmol/L (2.2-2.6)
      Phosphate              0.74 mmol/L (0.8-1.5)
      alkaline phosphatase   450 IU/L (50-110)
    ```

    Which one of the following investigations is most likely to help establish the diagnosis?

    A. 1,25-OH vitamin D levels
    B. 25-OH vitamin D levels
    C. Myeloma screen
    D. PTH level
    E. Sestamibi scan

4. **A 22-year-old university student was reviewed in the endocrine clinic with incidentally-detected elevated calcium level of 2.7 mmol/L. PTH levels were high normal. There was a strong family history of hypercalcaemia. Based on the urinary calcium creatinine excretion of <0.01, a diagnosis of familial hypocalciuric hypercalcaemia (FHH) was confirmed.**

    Which one of the following is a correct statement regarding FHH?

    A. Associated with nephrolithiasis
    B. Autosomal recessive inheritance
    C. PTH levels are usually low
    D. Results from activating mutation of calcium sensing receptor (CaSR)
    E. There is increased tubular calcium and magnesium reabsorption

5. **A 58-year-old solicitor was incidentally detected to have elevated calcium levels after routine blood tests as part of annual medical check-up. He had no medical problems in the past and was not taking any regular medications.**

```
Investigations:
  Urea                        8.5 mg/dL (7-10)
  Creatinine                  62 µmol/L (60-115)
  corrected calcium           2.64 mmol/L (2.2-2.6)
  Phosphate                   1.28 mmol/L (0.8-1.5)
  PTH                         6.8 pmol/L (1.6-7.2)
  25 OH vitamin D             82.2 µg/L
  calcium creatinine ratio    <0.01
```

Which one of the following is the most appropriate management plan in his case?

A. Bisphosphonates

B. Cinacalcet

C. Conservative management

D. Elective parathyroidectomy

E. 25-OH vitamin D replacement

6. **A 45-year-old woman of Afro-Caribbean origin presented to the medical assessment unit with symptoms of excessive thirst, nausea, increased frequency of micturition, and arthralgia after returning from a recent holiday in Egypt. She also had a long-standing history of a dry cough, which showed no improvement despite stopping Ramipril tablets that she was taking for blood pressure control. Her general physical and systemic examination is unremarkable except for having a tanned skin.**

```
Blood test results:
  Urea              8.5 mg/dL (5-10)
  Creatinine        105 µmol/L (60-115)
  Calcium           2.78 mmol/L (2.2-2.6)
  Phosphate         1.22 mmol/L (0.8-1.5)
  PTH               0.2 pmol/L (1.6-7.2)
  fasting glucose   4.5 mmol/L
```

Considering her history and clinical profile, which one of the following is the probable diagnosis?

A. FHH

B. Multiple myeloma

C. Pre-DM

D. Primary hyperparathyroidism (1° HPT)

E. Sarcoidosis

7. **A 54-year-old woman was referred to the endocrine clinic by her primary care physician with lethargy, arthralgia, and insomnia, together with an elevated calcium level of 2.70 mmol/L. Her medications include simvastatin, bendroflumethiazide, and paracetamol.**

```
Investigations:
   Urea                11.2 mg/dL (5-10)
   Creatinine          104 µmol/L (60-115)
   adjusted calcium    2.70 mmol/L (2.2-2.6)
   Phosphate           1.22 mmol/L (0.8-1.5)
   PTH                 2.5 pmol/L (1.5-7.5)
   TFT                 normal
```

Which one of the following is the most appropriate next step in the management of her hypercalcaemia?

A. Cinacalcet
B. Elective parathyroidectomy
C. Multiple endocrine neoplasia-1 (MEN-1) syndrome screening
D. Multiple endocrine neoplasia-2 (MEN-2) syndrome screening
E. Stop bendroflumethiazide

8. **A 35-year-old man with a background history of manic depressive psychosis and Type 2 DM presented to his primary care physician with symptoms of polydipsia, polyuria, and abdominal pain. He was taking lithium and metformin.**

```
Investigations:
   Urea                8.5 mg/dL (5-10)
   Creatinine          96 µmol/L (60-115)
   adjusted calcium    2.75 mmol/L (2.2-2.6)
   Phosphate           1.04 mmol/L (0.8-1.5)
   PTH                 8.8 pmol/L (1.5-7.5)
   HbA₁C               49 mmol/mol
```

Which one of the following is a correct statement with regards to the impact of lithium on calcium haemostasis?

A. Decreased serum magnesium levels
B. Decreased serum total and ionized calcium levels
C. Increased parathyroid gland sensitivity to calcium
D. Increased urinary calcium excretion
E. Shift of the set-point of calcium-PTH curve to the right

9. **A 72-year-old retired matron was admitted to the medical assessment unit with weight loss and elevated calcium. She had a background history of hypertension and gout. She was on allopurinol, bendroflumethiazide, and ramipril tablets.**

```
Investigations:
  Hb                          9.6 g/L (12.0-14.5)
  mean corpuscular volume     85 (80-98)
  urea                        13.4 mg/dL (5-10)
  creatinine                  142 µmol/L (60-115)
  adjusted calcium            3.05 mmol/L (2.2-2.6)
  PTH                         <0.5 pmol/L (1.5-7.5)
  total protein               92 g/L
  albumin                     26 g/L (35-40)
```

Which one of the following is the most likely cause of her hypercalcaemia?

A. Drug-induced hypercalcaemia

B. FHH

C. Multiple myeloma

D. 1° HPT

E. Secondary hyperparathyroidism (2° HPT)

10. **A 72-year-old woman presented to the medical assessment unit with progressive fatigue, malaise, and weight loss. On examination, she was cachectic and had a palpable hard left supra-clavicular lymph node.**

```
Investigations:
  urea                 15.5 mg/dL (5-10)
  creatinine           232 µmol/L (60-115)
  adjusted calcium     3.32 mmol/L (2.2-2.6)
  PTH                  <0.1 pmol/L (1.5-7.5)
  albumin              22 g/L (35-40)
```

Which one of the following is a correct statement regarding hypercalcaemia seen in patients with malignancy?

A. Increased bone resorption may contribute to hypercalcaemia

B. Lymphoma is associated with reduced calcitriol levels

C. Osteolytic metastases are seen in majority of patients

D. PTH contributes to humoral hypercalcaemia

E. Serum PTH concentrations are typically high or high normal

11. **A 92-year-old woman was found collapsed on the floor by her carer after an overnight mechanical fall. She had a background history of hypertension, dyslipidaemia, and temporal arteritis. She was on amlodipine, ramipril, atorvastatin, and prednisolone therapy.**

```
Investigations:
  Na                  152 mmol/L (135-145)
  K                   6.1 mmol/L (3.5-5.5)
  urea                25.5 mg/dL (5-10)
  creatinine          355 µmol/L (60-115)
  adjusted calcium    2.85 mmol/L (2.2-2.6)
  creatine kinase     raised
```

Which one of the following metabolic changes is seen in the early phases of rhabdomyolysis?

A. Hypercalcaemia

B. Hyperuricaemia

C. Hypokalaemia

D. Hypophosphataemia

E. Metabolic alkalosis

12. **An 18-year-old university student developed traumatic paraplegia secondary to a road traffic accident about 6 months previously, requiring prolonged immobilization and a period of rehabilitation. She was undergoing regular physiotherapy and was on a gradual road to recovery, although her mobility was limited to a few steps. Her general physical and systemic examination was unremarkable.**

```
Investigations:
  urea                7.5 mg/dL (7-20)
  creatinine          65 µmol/L (60-115)
  corrected calcium   2.80 mmol/L (2.2-2.6)
  phosphate           0.85 mmol/L (0.8-1.5)
  PTH                 0.8 pmol/L (1.6-7.2)
  total protein       54 g/L (65-75)
```

Which one of the following is the most probable underlying aetiology for her hypercalcaemia?

A. Immobilization

B. Malignancy

C. Multiple myeloma

D. Primary hyperparathyroidism

E. Sarcoidosis

13. **A 52-year-old male presented with a 4-week history of polyuria, polydipsia, and left-sided abdominal pain. On examination, he was apyrexial. A 1.5-cm neck lump was palpable and had a firm consistency. There was no lymphadenopathy and systemic examination showed mild left renal angle tenderness.**

```
Investigations:
  urea         12.2 mg/dL (7-20)
  creatinine   110 µmol/L (60-115)
  calcium      3.92 mmol/L (2.2-2.6)
  phosphate    0.45 mmol/L (0.8-1.5)
  PTH          92 pmol/L (1.6-7.2)
  R glucose    6.0 mmol/L
  HbA1C        41 mmol/mol (<46)
```

Which one of the following is the most likely cause of his clinical and biochemical profile?

A. Diabetes mellitus

B. Metastatic tumour

C. Parathyroid carcinoma

D. 2° HPT

E. Tertiary hyperparathyroidism

14. A 44-year-old man was diagnosed with 1° HPT, based on the biochemistry results (elevated calcium, low phosphate and raised PTH levels). His parathyroid ultrasound images were as shown in Figure 3.1.

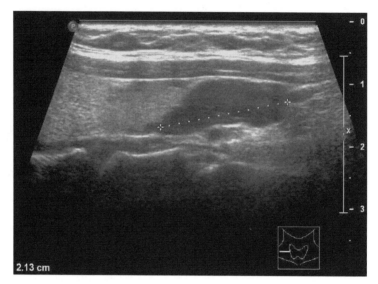

Figure 3.1 Ultrasound parathyroid gland

Reproduced with permission from Dr Nimit Goyal, Consultant Radiologist, Royal Gwent Hospital, Newport, UK

According to the summary statement from the 3rd International Workshop on the Management of Asymptomatic Primary Hyperparathyroidism, which one of the following is considered a valid indication for consideration for elective parathyroidectomy?

A. Age >50 years

B. Creatinine clearance <30 mL/min

C. Evidence of osteoporosis

D. Serum calcium >2.75 mmol/L

E. 24-hour urine calcium >50 mg/day

15. **A 32-year-old woman, with a background history of recently diagnosed 1° HPT, presented to the surgical assessment unit with acute left loin pain. On systemic examination, she had left renal angle tenderness.**

    ```
    Investigations:
      urea                7.1 mg/dL  (7-20)
      creatinine          76 µmol/L  (60-115)
      adjusted calcium    3.19 mmol/L (2.2-2.6)
      phosphate           0.78 mmol/L (0.8-1.5)
      PTH                 19.7 pmol/L (1.6-7.2)
      urine dipstick      + for ß-HCG and ++ blood.
    ```

    Her ultrasound abdomen confirmed a 17-week foetus, together with a 4-mm left renal angle calculus. On direct questioning, the patient confessed that the pregnancy was unplanned/unexpected, but she wanted to continue with it.

    Which one of the following is the most appropriate management approach for 1° HPT in her clinical scenario?

    A. Conservative management
    B. Elective parathyroidectomy in the post-partum period
    C. Elective parathyroidectomy in the second trimester
    D. Medical management with cinacalcet
    E. Medical management with zolendronate

16. **A 65-year-old retired school teacher was reviewed in the endocrine clinic due to elevated PTH levels. He had a background history of Type 2 DM and hypertension. Over the years, he had developed diabetic retinopathy, requiring laser therapy and nephropathy.**

    ```
    Investigations:
      urea                32.1 g/dL   (7-20)
      creatinine          226 µmol/L  (60-115)
      adjusted calcium    2.19 mmol/L (2.2-2.6)
      phosphate           1.78 mmol/L (0.8-1.5)
      PTH                 12.7 pmol/L (1.6-7.2)
    ```

    Which one of the following factors contributes to the development of 2° HPT in chronic kidney disease (CKD)?

    A. Calcium retention
    B. Increased calcitriol levels
    C. Increased conversion to 1,25 dihydroxy vitamin D
    D. Increased expression of vitamin D receptors on the parathyroid glands
    E. Phosphate retention

17. **A 33-year-old teacher underwent an elective parathyroidectomy for 1° HPT. Her post-operative stay in the hospital was uneventful and she was discharged home on day 3. On day 5 postoperatively, she noticed tingling around her face, with spasms in hands and was re-admitted to the hospital.**

```
Investigations:
  corrected calcium level  2.02 mmol/L (2.2-2.6)
  serum phosphate          0.6 mmol/L (0.8-1.5)
```

As a result she was commenced on oral calcium supplements. On day 7 post-operatively, symptoms recurred and a further fall in calcium level was noticed.

```
  corrected calcium level  1.89 mmol/L (2.2-2.6)
  serum phosphate          0.46 mmol/L (0.8-1.5)
```

She was started on IV calcium gluconate and alfacalcidol.

Which one of the following is the probable aetiology for her persistent hypocalcaemia?

A. Hungry bone syndrome

B. Hypoalbuminaemia

C. Iatrogenic hypoparathyroidism (post-surgery)

D. Malabsorption (coeliac disease)

E. Vitamin D deficiency

18. **A 32-year-old woman developed paraesthesia and carpo-pedal spasms during the post-operative period of an elective parathyroidectomy for 1° HPT. Based on her clinical profile and biochemistry results, a provisional diagnosis of hungry bone syndrome was made and she was started on alfacalcidol therapy.**

All of the following are known predictive factors for the development of hungry bone syndrome in patients undergoing elective parathyroidectomy except?

A. Larger volume of resected parathyroid adenoma

B. Older age group

C. Pre-operative alkaline phosphate level

D. Pre-operative 1,25 (OH)2 vitamin D level

E. Pre-operative PTH levels

19. **A 65-year-old South Asian woman with background history of Type 2 diabetes, hypertension, osteoporosis, and dyslipidaemia presented to her GP with lethargy, malaise, and generalized body aches.**

```
Investigations:
   urea          7.0 mg/dL (7-12)
   creatinine    66 µmol/L (60-115)
   calcium       2.28 mmol/L (2.2-2.6)
   phosphate     0.94 mmol/L (0.8-1.5)
   PTH           10.2 pmol/L (1.6-7.2)
```

Which one of the following investigations should be arranged to establish her underlying diagnosis?

A. Estimated glomerular filtration rate (eGFR)

B. 1, 25 (OH)2 vitamin D levels

C. PTH-related peptide

D. Sestamibi scan

E. 25-OH vitamin D levels

20. **An 86-year-old woman with a background history of ischaemic heart disease, congestive cardiac failure, and severe osteoporosis (previous fragility fractures), was incidentally detected to have 1° HPT, based on the following blood test results.**

```
Blood test results:
   urea          7.8 mg/dL (7-12)
   creatinine    92 µmol/L (60-115)
   calcium       2.89 mmol/L (2.2-2.6)
   phosphate     0.66 mmol/L (0.8-1.5)
   PTH           14.4 pmol/L (1.6-7.2)
```

In view of her multiple co-morbidities, she was deemed as not being a suitable candidate for elective parathyroidectomy and a decision was made to treat her medically with cinacalcet tablets.

Which one of the following best describes the mechanism of action of cinacalcet?

A. Decreases calcium reabsorption via the gastrointestinal tract

B. Increases calcium excretion by acting at the distal renal tubules

C. Increases calcium excretion by acting at the loop of Henlé

D. Increases sensitivity of calcium-sensing receptors on the parathyroid gland

E. Stimulates the parathyroid gland

21. **A 22-year-old university student was referred to the endocrine clinic with a recent history of fragility fracture. He had no significant past medical history and was on no medication. On examination, he had a BMI of 22 kg/m², with sparse facial and axillary hair growth. His systemic examination was unremarkable.**

    Which one of the following investigations may be useful in establishing the aetiology of his fragility fractures?

    A. Calcitonin level
    B. DEXA bone densitometry scan
    C. fracture risk assessment tool scoring
    D. IGF1 and IGFBP levels
    E. Testosterone and gonadotrophin levels

22. **A 66-year-old woman with end-stage renal failure due to diabetic nephropathy, was reviewed in the endocrine clinic with regards to her elevated PTH levels.**

    ```
    Blood results:
       urea         27.8 mg/dL  (7-12)
       creatinine   453 µmol/L  (60-115)
       calcium      2.25 mmol/L (2.2-2.6)
       phosphate    1.52 mmol/L (0.8-1.5)
       PTH          35.5 pmol/L (1.6-7.2)
    ```

    According to NICE guidelines, which one of the following statement is true regarding cinacalcet use in patients with 2° HPT due to end-stage renal failure in whom elective parathyroidectomy is contraindicated?

    A. Refractory 2° HPT with PTH > 25 pmol/L and high adjusted calcium
    B. Refractory 2° HPT with PTH > 25 pmol/L and low adjusted calcium
    C. Refractory 2° HPT with PTH > 85 pmol/L and high adjusted calcium
    D. Refractory 2° HPT with PTH > 85 pmol/L and low adjusted calcium
    E. Refractory 2° HPT with PTH > 100 pmol/L and low adjusted calcium

23. **A 75-year-old male with a background history of Type 2 diabetes for 30 years, CKD stage 5, and ischaemic heart disease was under regular review by the diabetic and renal physicians. He was on thrice weekly maintenance haemodialysis. In view of his progressive 2° HPT, he was started on cinacalcet therapy.**

    According to NICE guidelines, which one of these statements is true regarding cinacalcet use in 2° HPT?

    A. Cinacalcet should be continued for at least 6 months prior to assessing the response
    B. Cinacalcet should be only continued if there is reduction in intact PTH levels of >30% at 6 weeks
    C. Cinacalcet should be only continued if there is reduction in intact PTH levels of >30% at 4 months
    D. It should be only continued if there is reduction in intact PTH levels of >60% at 4 months
    E. It should be only continued if there is reduction in intact PTH levels of >60% at 6 months

24. **A 75-year-old woman with severe osteoporosis was referred to the endocrine clinic for consideration of denosumab therapy, as she had been intolerant to bisphosphonates in the past. She had no history of fragility fractures, and was on regular calcium and vitamin D supplements.**

    According to the NICE guidelines, what are the independent clinical risk factors that should be considered in assessing suitability for the use of denosumab in primary prevention of osteoporotic fragility fracture in post-menopausal women who are intolerant to bisphosphonate therapy?

    A. Alcohol (>4 units/day), diabetes, and 2° HPT
    B. Alcohol (>4 units/day), parental h/o hip fracture, and rheumatoid arthritis
    C. Diabetes, hypothyroidism, and 2° HPT
    D. Diabetes, rheumatoid arthritis, and smoking
    E. Hypothyroidism, parental h/o hip fracture, and smoking

25. **A 72-year-old woman with a previous history of fragility fractures and severe osteoporosis was being considered for denosumab therapy as she could not tolerate bisphosphonates.**

    Which one of the following correctly describes the mechanism of action of denosumab?

    A. It binds to the receptor activator of nuclear factor kappa β (RANK) ligand and prevents osteoclast formation thus leading to decreased bone resorption
    B. It binds to RANK ligand and stimulates osteocytes
    C. It binds to RANK ligand and stimulates the formation of osteoblasts, thus promoting bone growth
    D. It binds to the hepatic receptors and stimulates the secretion of growth factors
    E. It stimulates osteoblasts and inhibits osteoclasts directly

26. **A 56-year-old post-menopausal woman was referred to the endocrine clinic for further management of her severe osteoporosis, in view of her intolerance to bisphosphonate therapy. She was known to have hypertension and dyslipidaemia, and had recently sustained a fragility fracture. She was a smoker with a 25-pack year history and did not drink alcohol. There was no relevant family history. Her recent bone density scan showed T scores of –2.5 to –3.0 at the hip and lumbar spine.**

    According to NICE guidelines, which one of the following statement is true regarding strontium ranelate in her clinical scenario?

    A. Blood pressure needs to be controlled prior to strontium therapy
    B. She does not meet the criteria and she should be only given this medication if her T score is <–4.0
    C. She does not meet the criteria as strontium is only offered to patients aged >60
    D. She has to stop smoking before being considered for strontium therapy
    E. She should be given strontium as her T score is <–2.5

27. **A 67-year-old woman presented to the endocrine clinic for management of her osteoporosis. She had history of fragility fractures 5 years ago and had been on alendronic acid (70 mg/week) since then with good compliance. She had another non-traumatic fracture 3 months previously at L3. On examination, she had no features of Cushing's disease and was clinically euthyroid. Her TFTs, calcium, and vitamin D level were within normal range. A bone density scan showed a T score of –3.7 and –3.5 at the hip and spine, respectively.**

    Which one of the following is the most appropriate next step in her management?

    A. Continue alendronate
    B. Continue alendronate and add strontium
    C. Switch to raloxifene
    D. Switch to teriparatide
    E. Switch to zoledronic acid

28. **A 62-year-old man was referred to the osteoporosis clinic for advice on further management. He was known to have severe chronic obstructive airway disease and had been on oral prednisolone (20–30 mg/day) for the last 4 months. His calcium, TFTs, 25-hydroxy vitamin D levels, and serum testosterone levels were within the normal range.**

    His recent bone density scan showed T scores between –1.3 and –1.8 at hip and lumbar spine, respectively.

    Which one of the following is the most appropriate management approach in his case, based on National Osteoporosis Society (United Kingdom) guidelines?

    A. Alendronate
    B. Calcium and 25-hydorxy vitamin D supplement
    C. Denosumab
    D. No treatment
    E. Raloxifene

29. **A 56-year-old woman was seen in the osteoporosis clinic for further advice and management. She had a background history of breast cancer, which was treated with mastectomy, followed by aromatase inhibitor anastrozole. Her investigations, including full blood count, bone profile, 25-hydroxy vitamin D levels, TFTs, and liver and renal function tests were within normal range. A bone scan showed T scores of –2.1 and –2.4 at the hip and spine, respectively.**

    According to the consensus position statement from the UK expert group on bone loss in early breast cancer in post-menopausal women, which one of the following is the most appropriate approach in treating this patient?

    A. Bisphosphonates
    B. Calcium and vitamin D supplements
    C. Denosumab
    D. No medication
    E. Raloxifene

30. **A 36-year-old nurse was reviewed in the endocrinology clinic due to hypercalcaemia, despite undergoing a right inferior parathyroidectomy 10 months previously for a benign solitary parathyroid adenoma. She was currently not on any medication. She was a non-smoker with 3–4 units of alcohol consumption every week.**

    ```
    Biochemistry results:
      corrected calcium  2.85 mmol/L (2.2-2.6)
      phosphate          0.65 mmol/L (0.8-1.5)
      PTH                18.6 pmol/L (1.6-7.2)
    ```

    Which one of the following investigations can be useful in establishing the underlying aetiology for her recurrent hypercalcaemia?

    A. Amylase
    B. Bone scan
    C. CT of the abdomen and thorax
    D. Fasting gut hormone profile
    E. Sestamibi scan

31. A 46-year-old man presented to the clinic with a slowly progressive swelling and deformities of the hands. He had a history of Type 1 diabetes for the last 35 years and had been on haemodialysis for the last 4 years for diabetic nephropathy-induced end-stage renal failure. On examination, his digits of the hands were swollen and deformed, with no features of acute inflammation or infection.

```
Investigations:
   urea                52.5 mg/dL  (7-20)
   creatinine          474 µmol/L  (60-115)
   corrected calcium   3.36 mmol/L (2.2-2.6)
   phosphate           0.58 mmol/L (0.8-1.5)
   PTH                 36.8 pmol/L (1.6-7.2)
```

He underwent X-ray of the hands (see Figure 3.2).

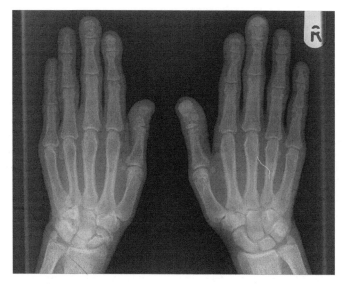

Figure 3.2 X-ray of the hands (AP view)

Which one of the following is the most appropriate approach to manage his hyperparathyroidism?

A. Alendronate (weekly)

B. Cinacalcet

C. Denosumab

D. Elective parathyroidectomy

E. Steroids

32. **A 55-year-old woman was referred to the endocrine clinic with a long-standing history of nausea, arthralgia, and malaise. She was known to have Type 2 diabetes and end-stage renal failure. She was on long-term haemodialysis therapy.**

```
Blood test results:
   Na                    140 mmol/L (135-145)
   K                     5.1 mmol/L (3.5-5.5)
   urea                  60.8 mg/dL (7-20)
   creatinine            501 µmol/L (60-115)
   corrected calcium     3.45 mmol/L (2.2-2.6)
   phosphate             1.06 mmol/L (0.8-1.5)
   PTH                   35.5 pmol/L (1.6-7.2)
```

Which one of the following is a characteristic finding, occasionally seen on clinical examination in patients with tertiary hyperparathyroidism and calciphylaxis?

A. Band keratopathy
B. Corneal ulcer
C. Dermal plaques
D. Tendon calcification
E. Xanthelasma

33. **A 25-year-old policeman was reviewed in the endocrinology clinic with recurrent hypercalcaemia. He had an elective left superior parathyroidectomy 10 months previously for a benign solitary parathyroid adenoma. He was not on any regular medication. His younger sister had recently been diagnosed with hypercalcaemia due to parathyroid gland hyperplasia. His general physical and systemic examination was normal.**

```
Biochemistry results:
   corrected calcium   2.92 mmol/L (2.2-2.6)
   phosphate           0.88 mmol/L (0.8-1.5)
   PTH                 17.5 pmol/L (1.6-7.2)
```

All of the following statements regarding MEN Type 1 syndrome are correct except?

A. Almost 100% penetrance by the age of 50 years
B. Hypercalcaemia is often detected on opportunistic screening
C. Presents usually between 2nd to 4th decade
D. Recurrence of disease may be seen
E. Relatively more common in men

34. **A 36-year-old schoolteacher was reviewed in the endocrinology clinic due to recurrent hypercalcaemia. She had right inferior parathyroidectomy 6 months previously for a benign solitary parathyroid adenoma. She was on omeprazole 40 mg/day for possible gastro-oesophageal reflux disease diagnosed by her primary care physician.**

```
Biochemistry results:
   corrected calcium  2.96 mmol/L (2.2-2.6)
   phosphate          0.89 mmol/L (0.8-1.5)
   PTH                19.5 pmol/L (1.6-7.2)
```

Which one of the following is the commonest gastro-enteropancreatic tumour seen in MEN-1 syndrome?

A. Gastrinoma
B. Glucaganoma
C. Insulinoma
D. Somatostatinoma
E. VIPoma

35. **A 23-year-old office clerk was referred to the thyroid clinic with a lump in the neck, which moved with swallowing. On examination, a 2-cm nodule was palpable on the right side of the thyroid with regional lymphadenopathy.**

```
Blood test results:
   adjusted calcium   2.86 mmol/L (2.2-2.6)
   phosphate          0.82 mmol/L (0.8-1.5)
   PTH                11.6 pmol/L (1.6-7.2)
```

Thyroid FNAC is suggestive of a diagnosis of medullary thyroid cancer.

Which one of the following genetic syndromes is associated with a medullary thyroid cancer?

A. Cowden's syndrome
B. McCune–Albright syndrome
C. Schmidt's syndrome
D. Sipple's syndrome (MEN-2a)
E. Wermer syndrome (MEN-1)

36. **A 19-year-old university student was referred to the thyroid clinic due to a recently noticed neck lump. On examination, a 2-cm thyroid nodule was palpable with evidence of cervical lymphadenopathy and mucosal neuromas on the tongue. FNAC confirmed the diagnosis of MTC. A clinical suspicion of MEN-2 was raised based on her clinical profile.**

    Which one of the following is a correct statement with regards to MEN-2 syndrome?

    A. Bilateral parathyroid hyperplasia is very common
    B. MTC in MEN-2B is less aggressive than in MEN-2A
    C. Prophylactic thyroidectomy is indicated in affected kindred <1 year of age in certain genotypes
    D. Pheochromocytoma is the commonest tumour in MEN-2
    E. There is no genotype–phenotype relationship with regards to MTC in MEN syndromes

37. **A 16-year-old student presented to the medical admission unit with spasms of hands along with twitching around the mouth. On examination, she had a BMI of 15 kg/m². Her general physical and systemic examination was unremarkable except for pallor and dental caries. She had prolonged QT interval on ECG.**

    ```
    Blood test results:
      adjusted calcium   1.84 mmol/L (2.2-2.6)
      phosphate          0.77 mmol/L (0.8-1.5)
      PTH                9.6 pmol/L (1.6-7.2)
      25-OH vitamin D    very low
    ```

    Which one of the following is the most appropriate treatment approach in her case?

    A. Cholecalciferol
    B. Ergocalciferol
    C. Intravenous calcium
    D. Oral phosphate supplementation
    E. Oral vitamin D 800 IU/day

38. **A 78-year-old man was admitted to the acute medical admission unit with 2 days history of feeling generally unwell, nausea, and repeated bouts of vomiting. He had been complaining of low back pain for the last 6 months for which he had taken analgesics. He had a background history of renal cell carcinoma, which required left nephrectomy 3 years ago. On examination, he was clinically dehydrated and systemic examination showed a 2-cm hepatomegaly.**

```
Blood test results:
   urea         22.5 mg/dL (7-12)
   creatinine   148 µmol/L (60-115)
   calcium      3.75 mmol/L (2.2-2.6)
```

Which one of the following is the most appropriate step for the immediate management of his acute hypercalcaemia?

A. Cinacalcet

B. Dexamethasone

C. Intravenous fluids

D. Intravenous pamidronate

E. Oral alendronate

39. **A 26-year-old woman presented to the medical assessment unit with cramps in her arms and legs. She had no significant past medical history and not on any regular medication. Her systemic examination was unremarkable and the blood pressure was 112/76 mmHg.**

```
Blood test results:
   Na                            135 mmol/L (135-45)
   K                             2.9 mmol/L (3.5-5.5)
   adjusted calcium              2.30 mmol/L (2.2-2.6)
   phosphate                     0.92 mmol/L (0.8-1.5)
   magnesium                     0.5 mmol/L (0.7-1)
   bicarbonate                   30 mEq/L (22-5)
   urine chloride excretion      normal
   plasma renin activity (PRA)   high
```

Which one of the following is the most likely diagnosis based on her clinical profile?

A. Apparent mineralocorticoid excess

B. Bartter's syndrome

C. Gitleman's syndrome

D. Liddle's syndrome

E. Renal tubular acidosis type 2

40. **A 66-year-old man presented to the clinic with a worsening of his lower back and right leg pain. There was no history of trauma or weight loss. On examination, he was mildly tender in the thoracolumbar region and had features of sensorineural hearing loss. His neurological system examination was normal. His right leg X-ray showed sclerotic changes as well as tibial deformity.**

```
Blood tests:
   adjusted calcium      2.36 mmol/L (2.2-2.6)
   phosphate             0.99 mmol/L (0.8-1.5)
   PTH                   4.4 pmol/L (1.6-7.2)
   alkaline phosphatase  450 IU/L (50-110)
```

Which one of the following is the most likely diagnosis based on his clinical profile?

A. Chondrosarcoma
B. Giant cell tumour of the bone
C. Paget's disease
D. Renal osteodystrophy
E. X-linked hypophosphatemia

41. **A 75-year-old man presented to clinic with a deformity of his tibia. He had no history of any recent trauma or injury. His bloods test results showed raised alkaline phosphatase with normal calcium and phosphate levels. His skull and spinal X-rays confirmed the diagnosis of Paget's disease.**

Which one of the following is the most appropriate treatment for this condition?

A. IV pamidronate
B. IV zolendronate
C. Oral calcium carbonate
D. Oral risedronate
E. Strontium

42. **An 18-year-old student presented to the medical admissions unit with twitching of the facial muscles and generalized muscle cramps. He had been on calcitriol supplementation since childhood. On physical examination, he was of short stature, with a raised BMI of 32 kg/m². He also had dental hypoplasia and small metacarpals.**

```
Blood tests results:
  adjusted calcium  1.96 mmol/L (2.2-2.6)
  phosphate         1.99 mmol/L (0.8-1.5)
  PTH               24.4 pmol/L (1.6-7.2)
```

Which one of the following is the most likely diagnosis based on his clinical profile?

A. Albright's hereditary osteodystrophy
B. Primary hyperparathyroidism
C. Pseudo pseudo-hypoparathyroidism
D. 2° HPT
E. Tertiary hyperparathyroidism

43. **A 32-year-old woman presented to the medical admission unit with a 3-day history of productive cough, fever, and bilious vomiting. She was known to have autoimmune hypothyroidism for which she was taking 75 µg/day of levothyroxine. She had a family history of pernicious anaemia and DM type 1. On examination, she was febrile, tachycardic (pulse rate: 121/min), and hypotensive (blood pressure: 86/48 mmHg). She had right basal crepitations and her chest X-ray revealed right basal atelectasis. Her capillary blood sugar was noted to be 3.1 mmol/L.**

```
Blood tests:
  Na                130 mmol/L (135-45)
  K                 5.7 mmol/L (3.5-5.5)
  urea              22.5 mg/dL (7-20)
  creatinine        129 µmol/L (60-115)
  adjusted calcium  2.80 mmol/L (2.2-2.6)
  phosphate         1.09 mmol/L (0.8-1.5)
  TSH               6.4 mU/L (0.35-5.5)
  free T4           12.5 pmol/L (11.5-22.7)
```

She was given intravenous fluids and broad spectrum antibiotics.

Which one of the following is the most appropriate next step in her management, pending the other blood results?

A. Bisphosphonates
B. Check PTH levels
C. Cinacalcet
D. Glucocorticoids
E. Increase levothyroxine dose

44. **An 18-year-old female Iranian migrant presented to the acute medical unit with spasms in the hands and legs. She was known to have oral candidiasis, for which she was on fluconazole. She had menarche at the age of 16 years and had irregular menses since then.**

```
Investigations:
  adjusted calcium   1.96 mmol/L (2.2-2.6)
  phosphate          1.69 mmol/L (0.8-1.5)
  PTH                0.2 pmol/L (1.6-7.2)
  FSH                56 IU/L (5-15)
  LH                 35 IU/L (5-15)
  oestrogen          <100 IU/L
```

Based on her clinical profile, which one of the following is the most likely diagnosis?

A. Albright's syndrome
B. Autoimmune polyglandular syndrome type I
C. Di-George syndrome
D. Sipple's syndrome
E. Wermer syndrome

45. **An 18-year-old Jamaican immigrant was admitted with gradually increasing leg weakness. He had sustained multiple fractures of his weight-bearing bones as a growing child and had suffered from bone pain at multiple sites in the past. His brother had similar bone-related symptoms. On examination, he was of short stature with bilateral bowing of femur and tibia.**

```
Investigations:
  adjusted calcium       2.36 mmol/L (2.2-2.6)
  phosphate              0.39 mmol/L (0.8-1.5)
  PTH                    6.8 pmol/L (1.6-7.2)
  25-OH vitamin D        normal
  alkaline phosphatase   350 IU/L (50-110)
```

His spinal MRI showed evidence of enthesopathy, especially involving the longitudinal ligaments of the spinal canal causing cord compression at the lumbar level.

Which one of the following is the most likely diagnosis based on his clinical profile?

A. Fanconi syndrome
B. Oncogenic osteomalacia
C. Paget's disease of the bone
D. Vitamin D deficiency
E. X-linked hypophosphataemia

1. E. Development of the parathyroid glands occurs from the fifth to seventh week of gestation. The superior glands arise from the fourth branchial pouch and have a short line of embryological descent, whereas the inferior glands arise from the third branchial pouch (together with the thymus) and have a longer embryological descent, which explains increased variability in their anatomical position.

PTH is a polypeptide hormone containing 84 amino-acids. Other peptide hormones include GH, ACTH, prolactin, anti-diuretic hormone (ADH), leptin, insulin, and somatostatin.

Renal absorption of calcium is enhanced by PTH at the ascending loop, loop of Henlé, and distal tubule. PTH reduces the reabsorption of phosphate at the proximal tubule via the sodium-phosphate co-transporter. 25-hydroxy vitamin D is the main storage form and the best measure of vitamin D status.

Akerström G, Malmaeus J, Bergström R. Surgical anatomy of human parathyroid glands. Surgery, 1984; 95(1): 14.

2. C. The demands of foetal growth lead to an adaptation of maternal homeostasis to provide the required calcium. Changes in maternal calcium regulation begin in the first trimester. Although total serum calcium falls, due to the haemodilution of the protein-bound fraction, the ionized and protein corrected components are unchanged.

Ardawi MS, Nasrat HA, BA'Aqueel HS. Calcium-regulating hormones and parathyroid hormone-related peptide in normal human pregnancy and postpartum: a longitudinal study. European Journal of Endocrinology, 1997; 137(4): 402–409.

Gertner JM, Coustan DR, Kliger AS, et al. Pregnancy as state of physiologic absorptive hypercalciuria. American Journal of Medicine, 1986; 81(3): 451–456.

3. D. The most likely cause of hypercalcaemia in this case is 1° HPT. The annual incidence is approximately 1 in 1000 and is commonly seen in post-menopausal women. The underlying aetiology of 1° HPT is parathyroid adenoma (80–85%) followed by parathyroid hyperplasia (~10–14%). Measuring PTH level is the first step in investigating hypercalcaemia.

Wermers RA, Khosla S, Atkinson EJ, et al. Incidence of primary hyperparathyroidism in Rochester, Minnesota, 1993–2001: an update on the changing epidemiology of the disease. Journal of Bone Mineral Research, 2006; 21(1): 171–177.

4. E. FHH is a benign condition, characterized by mild hypercalcaemia, and either high normal or slightly elevated PTH levels. It results from inactivation of the calcium sensing receptor gene (*CaSR*) and has an autosomal dominant inheritance with high penetrance. Urinary calcium excretion is typically low in this condition and calcium creatinine ratio is usually <0.01. The majority of patients do not have any symptoms/complications of hypercalcaemia due to the mild nature of it, although very rarely pancreatitis or chondrocalcinosis has been reported.

It is important to differentiate this from 1° HPT as the management varies (FHH—conservative). Parathyroidectomy is neither indicated nor curative in most cases of typical FHH. Atypical cases in both groups (FHH and 1° HPT) may rarely occur.

Christensen S, Nissen PH, Vestergaard P, et al. Discriminative power of three indices of renal calcium excretion for the distinction between familial hypocalciuric hypercalcaemia and primary hyperparathy-roidism: a follow-up study on methods. Clinical Endocrinology (Oxford), 2008; 69(5): 713–720.

Law W Jr and Heath H 3rd. Familial benign hypercalcaemia (hypocalciuric hypercalcaemia). Clinical and pathogenetic studies in 21 families. Annals of Internal Medicine, 1985; 102(4): 511–519.

5. C. The diagnosis is likely to be FHH in view of mildly elevated calcium levels, normal PTH, and a decreased calcium creatinine ratio, which is suggestive of reduced urinary calcium excretion. The management of FHH is conservative as it is not associated with any end-organ damage in the majority of individuals.

Brown E. Clinical lessons from the calcium-sensing receptor. Nature Clinical Practice. Endocrinology & Metabolism, 2007; 3(2): 122–133.

6. E. Sarcoidosis is a multi-system granulomatous disorder of unknown aetiology. It has three or four times higher incidence in the Afro-Caribbean ethnic group as compared with Caucasian population. Most of the individuals present with symptoms of sarcoidosis in their second to fourth decade of life. Hypercalcaemia is seen in approximately 10–20% patients with sarcoidosis. Diagnosis is based on clinical and radiological findings, with histo-pathological detection of non-caseating granulomas. Angiotensin-converting enzyme (ACE) levels can be elevated although not diagnostic. Hypercalcaemia in sarcoidosis is secondary to excess extra-renal production of 1,25 (OH)2 vitamin D in the granulomata. The biochemistry usually reveals normal 25-OH vitamin D, elevated 1,25 (OH)2 vitamin D and suppressed PTH. Treatment is with high dose corticosteroids.

This patient has an unexplained dry cough, arthralgia, and hypercalcaemia, all of which point towards a multi-system disorder, i.e. possible sarcoidosis in this case.

Baughman R, Teirstein AS, Judson MA, et al. Clinical characteristics of patients in a case control study of sarcoidosis. Case Control Etiologic Study of Sarcoidosis (ACCESS) Research Group. American Journal of Respiratory Critical Care Medicine, 2001; 164(10 Pt 1): 1885–1889.

Iannuzzi MC, Rybicki BA, Teirstein AS. Sarcoidosis. New England Journal of Medicine, 2007; 357(21): 2153–2165.

7. E. Thiazide diuretics reduce urinary excretion of calcium and may lead to mild hypercalcaemia. Metabolic alkalosis associated with thiazide diuretic use is also associated with hypercalcaemia as a result of a pH-dependent increase in protein-bound calcium. The incidence of thiazide-induced hypercalcaemia increases with age. In a population-based study reported from Minnesota, the mean duration between initiation of the thiazide diuretic therapy and detection of hypercalcaemia was 6–7 years. The majority of the patients who had persistent hypercalcaemia after stopping thaizides, were found to have primary hyperparathyroidism.

Wermers R, Kearns AE, Jenkins GD, et al. Incidence and clinical spectrum of thiazide-associated hyper-calcaemia. American Journal of Medicine, 2007; 120(10): 911.e9.

8. E. Lithium decreases the urinary calcium, as well as magnesium excretion, thus causing mild hypercalcaemia and mild hypermagnesaemia. In a proportion of patients, lithium therapy is also associated with a shift of the set-point for the calcium-PTH curve to the right, leading to hyper-calcaemia, hypocalciuria, and hyperparathyroidism. This pattern of shift is similar to that seen in individuals with FHH albeit the site of action of lithium appears to be beyond the CaSR, at the intracellular level.

Caskey F and Pickett T. Disturbed calcium metabolism in a patient with bipolar disorder and impaired renal function. Nephrology Dialysis Transplantation, (2005) 20(8): 1752–1755.

Haden S, Stoll AL, McCormick S, et al. Alterations in parathyroid dynamics in lithium-treated subjects. Journal of Clinical Endocrinology & Metabolism, 1997; 82(9): 2844–2848.

Nordenstrom J, Strigård K, Perbeck L, et al. Hyperparathyroidism associated with treatment of manic-depressive disorders by lithium. European Journal of Surgery, 1992; 158(4): 207–211.

9. C. The hypercalcaemia associated with bendroflumethiazide is usually mild. The biochemistry does not suggest either 1° (associated with normal or elevated PTH levels) or 2° HPT (calcium should have been normal or low, together with elevated PTH levels). The age and presenting symptoms, together with biochemistry showing suppressed PTH levels, normocytic anaemia, reversal of albumin–globulin ratio, severe hypercalcaemia, and renal dysfunction are all pointers towards a possible diagnosis of multiple myeloma.

Kariyawasan C, Hughes DA, Jayatillake MM, et al. Multiple myeloma: causes and consequences of delay in diagnosis. Quarterly Journal of Medicine, 2007; 100(10): 635–640.

Kyle R, Gertz MA, Witzig TE, et al. Review of 1027 patients with newly diagnosed multiple myeloma. Mayo Clinic Proceedings, 2003; 78(1): 21–33.

10. A. Hypercalcaemia is one of the commonest metabolic disturbances associated with malignancy. The most common malignancies associated with hypercalcaemia include breast, lung, and haematological (e.g. multiple myeloma). Hypercalcaemia of malignancy is either due to increased mobilization of calcium from the bones or inadequate calcium clearance from the renal tract. The former is either due to the direct bone destruction caused by the tumour (seen in approximately 20% of patients with hypercalcaemia) or due to the circulating factors (seen in approximately 75% of patients), such as PTHrP or increased cytokine production. Patients with underlying lymphoma have elevated calcium levels due to increased production of calcitriol (1,25 (OH)2 vitamin D) by tumour cells.

Clines G and Guise T. Hypercalcaemia of malignancy and basic research on mechanisms responsible for osteolytic and osteoblastic metastasis to bone. Endocrine Related Cancer, 2005; 12(3): 549–583.

Stewart A. Clinical practice. Hypercalcemia associated with cancer. New England Journal of Medicine, 2005; 352(4): 373–379.

11. B. Hypocalcaemia occurs in the early phase of rhabdomyolysis because of an influx of calcium into the damaged myocytes, which is then deposited. Decreased bone responsiveness to the PTH has also been reported in patients with rhabdomyolysis.

Akmal M, Bishop JE, Telfer N, et al. Hypocalcemia and hypercalcemia in patients with rhabdomyolysis with and without acute renal failure. Journal of Clinical Endocrinology & Metabolism, 1986; 63(1): 137–142.

Llach F, Felsenfeld AJ, Haussler MR. The pathophysiology of altered calcium metabolism in rhabdomyolysis-induced acute renal failure. Interactions of parathyroid hormone, 25-hydroxycholecalciferol, and 1, 25-dihydroxycholecalciferol. New England Journal of Medicine, 1981; 305(3): 117–123.

12. A. Prolonged immobilization may result in hypercalcaemia, hypercalciuria, and osteoporosis. The parathyroid 1,25-dihydroxy vitamin D axis is suppressed in patients with immobilization-induced hypercalcaemia. A single dose of pamidronate (60 mg) has been reported to resolve the hypercalcaemia in almost 80% of patients with spinal cord injury and immobility.

Gilchrist N, Frampton CM, Acland RH, et al. Alendronate prevents bone loss in patients with acute spinal cord injury: a randomized, double-blind, placebo-controlled study. Journal of Clinical Endocrinology & Metabolism, 2007; 92(4): 1385–1390.

Massagli T and Cardenas D. Immobilization hypercalcemia treatment with pamidronate disodium after spinal cord injury. Archives of Physical Medicine and Rehabilitation, 1999; 80(9): 998.

Stewart A., Adler M, Byers CM, et al. Calcium homeostasis in immobilization: an example of resorptive hypercalciuria. New England Journal of Medicine, 1982; 306(19): 1136–1140.

13. C. The kidney function shown should not result in tertiary hyperparathyroidism. Parathyroid carcinoma is a rare cause of elevated PTH and calcium, accounting for <1% of patients with hyperparathyroidism. The major clinical manifestations of parathyroid carcinoma are:

- Mean age 44–54 years.
- Mean serum calcium concentration 3.7–4.0 mmol/L.
- Neck mass 34–52%.
- Bone disease 34–73%.
- Renal disease 30–70%.
- Pancreatitis 0–15%.

Left renal angle pain/tenderness in this patient could be due to nephrolithiasis.

Obara T and Fujimoto Y Diagnosis and treatment of patients with parathyroid carcinoma: an update and review. World Journal of Surgery, 1991; 15(6): 738–744.

Wynne A, van Heerden J, Carney JA, et al. Parathyroid carcinoma: clinical and pathologic features in 43 patients. Medicine (Baltimore), 1992; 71(4): 197–205.

14. C. Indications for surgery in asymptomatic primary hyperparathyroidism as per 3rd International Workshop (2008):

- Serum calcium >2.85 mmol/L.
- Age <50 years.
- Creatinine clearance <60 mL/min.
- T score <−2.5 at any site and/or previous fragility fracture.

Bilezikian J, Khan AA, Potts JT Jr, et al. Guidelines for the management of asymptomatic primary hyperparathyroidism: summary statement from the Third International Workshop. Journal of Clinical Endocrinology & Metabolism, 2009; 94: 335–339.

15. C. Severe hypercalcaemia during pregnancy may carry significant maternal and foetal risks. Maternal presentation may include hyperemesis, nephrolithiasis, recurrent urinary tract infections, and pancreatitis. Neonatal complications may include hypocalcaemia and tetany (secondary to foetal PTH suppression), preterm delivery, low birth weight, and foetal demise. Surgery during the second trimester is the preferred treatment for symptomatic patients; however, observation may be appropriate in patients with asymptomatic, mild hypercalcaemia.

McMullen T, Learoyd DL, Williams DC, et al. Hyperparathyroidism in pregnancy: options for localization and surgical therapy; World Journal of Surgery, 2010; 34(8): 1811–1816.

Schnatz P and Curry SL. Primary hyperparathyroidism in pregnancy: evidence-based management; Obstetrics and Gynecological Survey, 2002; 57(6): 365–376.

16. E. Progressive renal dysfunction results in hyperphosphataemia (due to reduced excretion of phosphate) and reduced calcitriol levels (due to reduced 1-hydroxylation). This ultimately results in hypocalcaemia. These abnormalities result in increased PTH levels via various mechanisms causing 2° HPT.

Levin A, Bakris GL, Molitch M et al. Prevalence of abnormal serum vitamin D, PTH, calcium, and phosphorus in patients with chronic kidney disease: results of the study to evaluate early kidney disease. Kidney International, 2007; 71(1): 31–38.

17. A. This woman likely would have had increased bone resorption due to increased osteoclastic activity, as a result of high PTH levels pre-operatively. Her post-operative hypocalcaemia and hypophosphataemia is probably due to the rapid uptake of calcium and phosphate by the bones, otherwise labelled as hungry bone syndrome.

Brasier A and Nussbaum SR. Hungry bone syndrome: clinical and biochemical predictors of its occurrence after parathyroid surgery. American Journal of Medicine, 1988; 84(4): 654–660.

Davenport A and Stearns M. Administration of pamidronate helps prevent immediate post-parathyroidectomy hungry bone syndrome. Nephrology (Carlton), 2007; 12: 386–390.

18. D. Sudden withdrawal of PTH causes an imbalance between osteoblast-mediated bone formation and osteoclast-mediated bone resorption, leading to a marked net increase in bone uptake of calcium, phosphate, and magnesium. Pre-operative urea nitrogen, alkaline phosphatase, PTH levels, older age, and volume of resected parathyroid adenoma have been shown to predict the development of hungry bone syndrome in patients undergoing elective parathyroidectomy.

Brasier A and Nussbaum SR. Hungry bone syndrome: clinical and biochemical predictors of its occurrence after parathyroid surgery. American Journal of Medicine, 1988; 84(4): 654–660.

19. E. This woman has elevated PTH in the presence of normal calcium levels suggestive of 2° HPT. Her kidney function is normal, ruling out renal impairment as a driving factor for elevated PTH levels. Vitamin D deficiency is one of the commonest reasons for 2° HPT. A level of 25 OH vitamin D <20 µg/L has been linked to 2° HPT and needs to be corrected prior to further assessment of elevated PTH in this scenario. 25 OH vitamin D is the main storage form and the best measure of vitamin D status.

Holick M. High prevalence of vitamin D inadequacy and implications for health. Mayo Clinic Proceedings 2006; 81:353–373.

20. D. By increasing the sensitivity of calcium sensing receptors on the parathyroid glands, it switches off the PTH secretion, thus decreasing the serum calcium levels.

Block G, Martin KJ, de Francisco AL, et al. Cinacalcet for secondary hyperparathyroidism in patients receiving hemodialysis. New England Journal of Medicine, 2004; 350(15): 1516–1525.

21. E. It is important to rule out secondary causes of osteoporosis in young adult men presenting with a history of fragility fractures. This young man presented with history of fragility fracture and the only thing of note on his examination was scanty facial and axillary hair growth, suggestive of delayed development of secondary sexual characteristics. His testosterone and gonadotrophin status needs to be assessed. See Table 3.1 for a list of conditions that can result in osteoporosis.

Table 3.1 List of conditions resulting in osteoporosis

Endocrine	Gastrointestinal	Genetic	Rheumatological	Haematological	Medications
Acromegaly	Anorexia nervosa	Turner's	Ankylosing spondylitis	Leukaemia	Antipsychotics
Cushing's syndrome	Coeliac disease	Haemochromatosis	Rheumatoid arthritis	Lymphoma	Retrovirals
Hypogonadism	Inflammatory bowel disease	Klinefelter's syndrome	Systemic lupus erythematosus	Metastatic disease	Heparin
Hyperparathyroidism	Malabsorption syndromes				Lithium
Prolactinoma	Primary biliary cirrhosis				Steroids
Thyrotoxicosis					
Type 1 diabetes					

Gennari L and Bilezikian J. Osteoporosis in men. Endocrinology & Metabolism Clinics of North America 2007; 36: 399–419.

22. C. Cinacalcet is recommended for the treatment of refractory 2° HPT in patients with end-stage renal disease (including those with calciphylaxis) only in those:

- Who have 'very uncontrolled' plasma levels of intact PTH (defined as greater than 85 pmol/L [800 pg/mL]) that are refractory to standard therapy, and a normal or high adjusted serum calcium level.
- Those in whom surgical parathyroidectomy is contraindicated, because the risks of surgery are considered to outweigh the benefits.

NICE. Cinacalcet for the treatment of secondary hyperparathyroidism in patients with end-stage renal disease on maintenance dialysis therapy. NICE Guideline TA 117. NICE, 2007.

23. C. Response to cinacalcet treatment should be monitored regularly and treatment should be continued only if a reduction in the plasma levels of intact PTH of 30% or more is seen within 4 months, including dose escalation as appropriate.

NICE. Cinacalcet for the treatment of secondary hyperparathyroidism in patients with end-stage renal disease on maintenance dialysis therapy. NICE Guideline TA 117. NICE, 2007.

24. B. Denosumab is recommended as the treatment option for the primary prevention of osteoporotic fragility fractures in post-menopausal women at increased risk of fractures only if:

- They are intolerant to bisphosphonate therapy or it is contraindicated
- In those who have a combination of T-score, age, and number of independent clinical risk factors for fracture as indicated in Table 3.2.

Table 3.2 T-scores (SD) at (or below) which denosumab therapy is recommended (for primary prevention) when bisphosphonates are not suitable or are contraindicated.

Age (in years)	Risk factors 0	Risk factors 1	Risk factors 2
65–69	–	–4.5	–4.0
70–74	–4.5	–4.0	–3.5
75 or more	–4.0	–4.0	–3.0

National Institute for Health and Clinical Excellence (2011) Adapted from 'TA204: Denosumab for the prevention of osteoporotic fractures in postmenopausal women'. Manchester: NICE. Available from http://guidance.nice.org.uk/TA204. Reproduced with permission. NICE has not checked to confirm that the book accurately reflects the original NICE publications, and no guarantees are given by NICE with regards to accuracy.

Independent clinical risk factors for fracture include a parental history of hip fracture, an alcohol intake of 4 or more units per day, and rheumatoid arthritis.

NICE. Denosumab for the prevention of osteoporotic fractures in postmenopausal women. NICE Guideline TA 204. NICE, 2010.

25. A. Denosumab binds to the cytokine RANK ligand, preventing it from binding to its receptor, RANK. It also prevents the maturation of osteoclast precursors and promotes apoptosis of mature and multinucleated osteoclasts, thus leading to reduced bone resorption.

Hanley D, Adachi JD, Bell A, et al. Denosumab: mechanism of action and clinical outcomes. International Journal of Clinical Practice, 2012 Dec; 66(12): 1139–1146.

26. B. Strontium ranelate and raloxifene are recommended as alternative treatment options for the secondary prevention of osteoporotic fragility fractures in postmenopausal women only if:

- They are unable to comply with the special instructions for the administration of alendronate and either risedronate or etidronate **or** have a contraindication to **or** are intolerant of alendronate, and either risedronate or etidronate.
- They have a combination of T-score, age, and number of independent clinical risk factors for fracture (parental history of hip fracture, alcohol intake of 4 or more units per day, and rheumatoid arthritis) as indicated in Table 3.3.

Table 3.3 T-scores (SD) at (or below) which denosumab therapy is recommended (for primary prevention) when bisphosphonates are not suitable/contra-indicated.

Age	Number of independent risk factors		
	0	1	2
50–54 years	Not recommended	−3.5	−3.5
55–59 years	−4.0	−3.5	−3.5
60–64 years	−4.0	−3.5	−3.5
65–69 years	−4.0	−3.5	−3.0
70–74 years	−3.0	−3.0	−2.5
75 years or older	−3.0	−2.5	−2.5

National Institute for Health and Clinical Excellence (2011) Adapted from 'TA161 Alendronate, etidronate, risedronate, raloxifene, strontium ranelate and teriparatide for the secondary prevention of osteoporotic fragility fractures in postmenopausal women'. Manchester: NICE. Available from http://guidance.nice.org. uk/TA161. Reproduced with permission. NICE has not checked to confirm that the book accurately reflects the original NICE publications, and no guarantees are given by NICE with regards to accuracy.

NICE. Alendronate, etidronate, risedronate, raloxifene, strontium ranelate and teriparatide for the secondary prevention of osteoporotic fragility fractures in postmenopausal women (amended). NICE guideline TA161. NICE, 2008.

27. D. Teriparatide is recommended as an alternative treatment option for the secondary prevention of osteoporotic fragility fractures in post-menopausal women:

- Who are unable to tolerate alendronate, and either risedronate or etidronate; **or** have a contraindication to alendronate and either risedronate or etidronate; **or** who have a contraindication to, or are intolerant of strontium ranelate; **or** who have had an unsatisfactory response to treatment with alendronate, risedronate or etidronate.
- Who are aged 65 years or older with a:
  - ◆ T score of −4.0 SD or below.
  - ◆ T score of −3.5 SD or below plus more than two fractures.
- Who are aged 55–64 years with a T score of −4 SD or below, plus more than two fractures.

Data from NICE guidelines (TA161) Alendronate, etidronate, risedronate, raloxifene, strontium ranelate and teriparatide for the secondary prevention of osteoporotic fragility fractures in postmenopausal women. Published 2011.

NICE. Alendronate, etidronate, risedronate, raloxifene, strontium ranelate and teriparatide for the secondary prevention of osteoporotic fragility fractures in postmenopausal women (amended). NICE guideline TA161. NICE, 2008.

28. A. Oral glucocorticoid use for 3 months or more in a patient <65 years of age warrants assessment of bone density by DEXA scan (at hip +/− spine) if there is no previous history of fragility fractures. A T score of −1.5 or less on DEXA scan is an indication to treat the patient with bisphosphonates beside use of general measures, such as regular exercise, tapering of steroid dose (if possible), and avoiding alcohol and tobacco use. Calcium and vitamin D therapy is used as an adjunct.

Bone and Tooth Society, National Osteoporosis Society, Royal College of Physicians. Glucocorticoid-induced osteoporosis: guidelines for prevention and treatment. RCP, 2002.

29. A. Women with breast cancer who have received chemotherapy, and are aged <75 years or without major risk factors, are categorized into three groups based on baseline bone mineral density (BMD assessment):

- High-risk group (a baseline T-score of <−2 at the lumbar spine or either hip): bisphosphonate therapy at osteoporosis doses in addition to lifestyle advise, and calcium and vitamin D supplementation.
- Medium-risk group (a T-score between −1 and −2): lifestyle advice plus calcium (1 g/day) and vitamin D (400–800 IU) supplementation are recommended, unless dietary intake of calcium exceeds 1 g/day and serum 25-hydroxy vitamin D is known to be >20 µg/L.
- Low-risk group (T-score >−1): the risk of developing osteoporosis over a 5-year treatment period is very low. Advice on lifestyle (diet, weight-bearing exercise, reduced alcohol consumption, and cessation of smoking) is sufficient and no specific intervention or follow-up assessment of BMD is required.

Data from Reid DM et al. Guidance for the management of breast cancer treatment-induced bone loss: a consensus position statement from a UK Expert Group. Cancer Treat Rev 2008; 34:S1–S18.

Reid DM, Doughty J, Eastell R, et al. Guidance for the management of breast cancer treatment-induced bone loss: a consensus position statement from a UK Expert Group. Cancer Treatment Reviews, 2008; 34: S1–S18.

30. D. MEN-1 is a rare hereditary endocrine syndrome (estimated incidence is 1 in 40000), characterized primarily by tumours of parathyroid glands (95% of cases), endocrine gastro-enteropancreatic tract (30–80% of cases), and anterior pituitary. It is inherited in the autosomal dominant manner. A diagnosis of MEN-1 syndrome should be considered in the following clinical scenarios:

- Recurrent primary hyperparathyroidism, despite previous parathyroid surgery.
- Parathyroid hyperplasia.
- Young patients with primary hyperparathyroidism.
- Family history of primary hyperparathyroidism.

Thakker R, Newey PJ, Walls GV, et al. Clinical practice guidelines for multiple endocrine neoplasia type 1 (MEN1). Journal of Clinical Endocrinology & Metabolism 2012; 97: 2990–3011.

31. D. This patient probably has tertiary hyperparathyroidism as evidenced by elevated calcium and PTH levels, in the presence of end-stage renal failure, together with the evidence of soft tissue calcification on hand X-ray. Elective parathyroidectomy remains the treatment of choice in patients with tertiary hyperparathyroidism.

National Kidney Foundation. K/DOQI clinical practice guidelines for bone metabolism and disease in chronic kidney disease. American Journal of Kidney Disease, 2003; 42:S1–S201.

32. A. Band keratopathy is occasionally seen in patients with metastatic calcification especially in the context of tertiary hyperparathyroidism, as in this patient. It involves calcium precipitation as a horizontal band across the central cornea. It is associated with reduced visual acuity and eye pain.

Klaassen-Broekema N, Van Bijsterveld OP. Limbal and corneal calcification in patients with chronic renal failure. British Journal of Ophthalmology, 1993; 77(9): 569–571.

33. E. The incidence of MEN-1 is equal in both sexes.

Thakker R, Newey PJ, Walls GV, et al. Clinical practice guidelines for multiple endocrine neoplasia type 1 (MEN1). Journal of Clinical Endocrinology & Metabolism 2012; 97: 2990–3011.

34. A. Various tumours seen in MEN-1 syndrome and their estimated penetrance by the age of 40 years are shown in Table 3.4.

Table 3.4 Prevalence of various endocrine neoplasia in MEN-1 syndrome

Parathyroid adenoma	90%
Enteropancreatic tumours: (60–70% overall)	
• gastrinoma	30–40%
• insulinoma	10%
• others (glucaganoma, vipoma, somatostatinoma)	2%
Anterior pituitary tumours: (10–20%)	
• prolactinoma (PRL)	20%
• GH	5%
• non-functioning	5%
• GH + PRL	5%
• ACTH/TSH	Rare

Brandi M, Gagel RF, Angeli A, et al. Guidelines for diagnosis and therapy of MEN type 1 and type 2. Journal of Clinical Endocrinology & Metabolism 2001; 86(12): 5658–5671.

35. D. Sipple's syndrome or MEN-2A is characterized by medullary thyroid cancer (>90%), pheochromocytoma (40–50%), primary parathyroid hyperplasia (10–20%), and very rarely cutaneous lichen amyloidosis. It is associated with a germline rearranged during transfection (RET) mutation. Men and women are affected in equal proportions due to autosomal dominant inheritance patterns.

American Thyroid Association Guidelines Task Force, Kloos R, Eng C et al. American Thyroid Association Guidelines Task Force, Medullary thyroid cancer: management guidelines of the American Thyroid Association. Thyroid, 2009; 19: 565–612.

Brandi M, Gagel RF, Angeli A, et al. Guidelines for diagnosis and therapy of MEN type 1 and type 2. Journal of Clinical Endocrinology & Metabolism 2001; 86(12): 5658–5671.

36. C. There is a strong correlation between genotype and phenotype in MEN with regards to MTC (see Table 3.5).

Table 3.5 Genotype in MTC and timing of surgery

Level of malignancy	RET genotype/mutation in codon number	Timing of surgery
Highest risk	883, 918, 804	<1 year of age
High	634	2–4 years
Moderate	609, 611, 618, 620, 630, 804	<6 years
Low	533, 649, 666, 768, 790, 791, 8040, 891, 912	<10 years

American Thyroid Association Guidelines Task Force, Kloos R, Eng C et al. American Thyroid Association Guidelines Task Force, Medullary thyroid cancer: management guidelines of the American Thyroid Association. Thyroid, 2009; 19: 565–612.

Skinner MA, Moley JA, Dilley WG, et al. Prophylactic thyroidectomy in multiple endocrine neoplasia type 2A. New England Journal of Medicine, 2005; 353: 1105–1113.

37. C. This young girl possibly suffers from anorexia nervosa in view of her very low BMI and clinical profile. There is evidence of vitamin D deficiency from the blood tests, which has possibly resulted in hypocalcaemia and 2° HPT. She also has evidence of prolonged QT interval on the ECG; hence, the need for urgent correction of calcium, which is better done by intravenous route.

Benoit S, Mendelsohn AB, Nourjah P, et al. Risk factors for prolonged QTc among US adults: Third National Health and Nutrition Examination Survey. European Journal of Cardiovascular Preventive Rehabilitation, 2005; 12(4): 363.

38. C. This gentleman has non-specific symptoms, such as nausea and vomiting, which are probably due to severe hypercalcaemia. He is clinically dehydrated, and needs immediate rehydration with intravenous fluids with careful monitoring of renal function and electrolytes. Bisphosphonates such as pamidronate (in a dose of 15–60 mg given slowly intravenously) should only be given once the patient is well hydrated. The likely cause of his severe hypercalcaemia is humoral hypercalcaemia (PTHrP mediated).

Bilezikian JP. Management of acute hypercalcemia. New England Journal of Medicine 1992; 326: 1196–1203.

39. C. Gitelman syndrome is an autosomal recessive disorder that presents with various metabolic abnormalities, including hypokalaemia, hypomagnesaemia, metabolic alkalosis, hypocalciuria, and normal blood pressure. Patients have mutations in the gene coding for the thiazide-sensitive Na/Cl co-transporter in the distal tubule. It is not usually diagnosed until late childhood or early adulthood. Clinical manifestations include arm and leg cramps (due to low K^+ and low Mg^{2+}), severe fatigue, polyuria/nocturia (due to salt and water loss), chondrocalcinosis (due to chronic hypomagnesaemia), and occasionally growth retardation. The diagnosis is mainly of exclusion. Treatment is largely supportive with a potassium-sparing diuretic, and with potassium chloride and magnesium supplementation. Surreptitious vomiting or diuretic abuse can mimic this. However, there was no suggestion in the history or physical examination of this. Moreover, her urinary chloride would be expected to be low in surreptitious vomiting/diuretic abuse in view of chronic hypochloraemia and hypovolaemia.

Cruz DN, Shaer AJ, Bia MJ, et al. Gitelman's syndrome revisited: an evaluation of symptoms and health-related quality of life; Yale Gitelman's and Bartter's Syndrome Collaborative Study Group. Kidney International 2001; 59(2): 710–717.

40. C. This patient presented with bone pain and hearing loss. The only main abnormality in his bloods was raised alkaline phosphatase. His X-ray of the right leg showed typical changes (sclerotic and deformed bones) associated with Paget's disease. Other radiological changes that may be seen include lytic, as well as sclerotic changes on skull X-ray, and densely sclerotic vertebral bodies.

van Staa TP, Selby P, Leufkens HG, et al, Incidence and natural history of Paget's disease of bone in England and Wales. Journal of Bone Mineral Research, 2002; 17(3): 465–471.

41. B. The prevalence of Paget's disease is about 2% over the age of 55 years in UK. Only 10% of these patients are symptomatic. The indications for treating Paget's disease include the presence of symptoms (pain), deformity, complications (such as deafness, spinal cord compression), and hypercalcaemia. Bisphosphonates form the mainstay of the treatment. The bisphosphonates licensed for the treatment in Paget's disease include pamidronate, risedronate, etidronate, tiludronic acid and zoledronate. Of these, zoledronate has the longest action and often only a single dose is required for treatment purposes.

Ralston SH, Langston AL, Reid IR. Pathogenesis and management of Paget's disease of bone. Lancet, 2008; 372: 155–163.

42. A. Pseudohypoparathyroidism (PHP) is a heterogeneous group of disorders characterized by hypocalcaemia, hyperphosphataemia and increased PTH levels due to the insensitivity to the PTH (see Table 3.6). The molecular defects in the gene (*GNAS1*) encoding the alpha-subunit of the stimulatory G protein contribute to at least three different forms of the disease: PHP type 1a, PHP type 1b, and pseudo-pseudohypoparathyroidism (pseudo-PHP).

Table 3.6 Characteristics of various types of pseudohypoparathyroidism

Condition	Appearance	Calcium	Phosphorus	PTH	Genetic imprinting
PHP 1A	Skeletal defects	Low	High	High	From mother
PHP 1B	Normal	Low	High	High	From mother
Pseudo-PHP	Skeletal defects	Normal	Normal	Normal	From father

Davies SJ, Hughes HE. Imprinting in Albright's hereditary osteodystrophy. Journal of Medical Genetics Feb 1993; 30(2): 101–103.

Shalitin S, Davidovits M, Lazar L, et al. Clinical heterogeneity of pseudohypoparathyroidism: from hyper- to hypocalcaemia. Hormone Research, 2008; 70(3): 137–144.

43. D. This patient with strong personal and family history of autoimmune diseases, presented with features of chest sepsis along with classical signs of adrenal insufficiency. Mildly raised TSH and hypercalcaemia are often seen in this context. Hypercalcaemia in this case might have been exacerbated by dehydration. The priority here is to give her intravenous glucocorticoids as soon as possible along with fluids (If possible, a blood sample should be sent for random cortisol levels before steroid therapy is started).

Burke CW. Adrenocortical insufficiency. Clinical Endocrinology & Metabolism 1985; 14: 947–976.

Zelissen PM, Bast EJ, Croughs RJ. Associated autoimmunity in Addison's disease. Journal of Autoimmunization 1995; 8: 121–130.

44. B. Autoimmune polyglandular syndrome type I (APS1), also referred to as the autoimmune polyendocrinopathy-candidiasis-ectodermal dystrophy (APECED) syndrome, is a rare autosomal recessive disorder. Females are more commonly affected than males. It is most common among Finns, Sardinians, and Iranian Jews. Clinical manifestations include hypoparathyroidism (~90%), mucocutaneous candidiasis (75%), adrenal insufficiency (60%), and primary hypogonadism (45%). Other manifestations include hypothyroidism, malabsorption syndromes, pernicious anaemia, and alopecia.

Ahonen P, Myllarniemi S, Sipila I, et al. Clinical variation of autoimmune polyendocrinopathy-candidiasis-ectodermal dystrophy (APECED) in a series of 68 patients. New England Journal of Medicine, 1990; 322(26): 1829–1836.

Alimohammadi M, Bjorklund P, Hallgren A, et al. Autoimmune polyendocrine syndrome type 1 and NALP5, a parathyroid autoantigen. New England Journal of Medicine, 2008; 358(10): 1018–1028.

Trence D, Morley JE, and Handwerger BS. Polyglandular autoimmune syndromes. American Journal of Medicine, 1984; 77(1): 107.

45. E. Vitamin D-resistant rickets (VDDR) used to be the term used for disorders that had hypophosphataemia and rickets, because they resemble vitamin D deficiency, but do not respond to the replacement of vitamin D in the expected manner. This entity involves a unique abnormality in the form of renal phosphate wasting, which is the primary problem. Most of the cases are X-linked (phosphate-regulating endopeptidase on the X chromosome). Clinical features include slow growth, deformity of the bones as weight-bearing starts, enthesopathy (particularly in adults), and dentin defects causing tooth abscess. Biochemically, there is hypophosphataemia, normal calcium, normal to high PTH, elevated alkaline phosphatase. Bone biopsy although not necessary for diagnosis, will show evidence of osteomalacia and hypomineralization. Treatment in children includes phosphate and calcitriol administration. Symptomatic adults will benefit from similar therapy.

Alizadeh Naderi AS and Reilly RF. Hereditary disorders of renal phosphate wasting. Nature Reviews Nephrology, 2010; 6: 657–665.

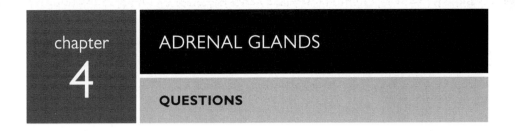

1. The adrenal gland is made up of two distinct layers—the cortex and medulla. The adrenal cortex is further sub-divided into three different layers:
    - zona glomerulosa
    - zona fasciculata
    - zona reticularis

    All of the following associations between the layer of adrenal gland and hormone secretion are correct except?

    A. Medulla—catecholamines
    B. Zona fasciculata—glucocorticoids and aldosterone
    C. Zona glomerulosa—aldosterone
    D. Zona reticularis—androstenedione
    E. Zona reticularis—dihydroepiandrostenedione and glucocorticoids

2. The secretion of various hormones from the adrenal gland is regulated by various hormones, extracellular fluid volume status, electrolyte levels, and cytokines.

    All of the following factors/hormones play a part in the regulation of synthesis and secretion of mineralocorticoids (aldosterone) from zona glomerulosa except?

    A. ACTH
    B. Adrenaline
    C. Angiotensin 2
    D. Atrial natriuretic peptide
    E. Potassium

3. Adrenal gland development starts at about week 6 of embryological development, with the cortex developing from mesoderm of the posterior abdominal wall, while the inner medulla is derived from neuroectoderm.

    Which one of the following statements regarding adrenal gland physiology and development is correct?

    A. Cholesterol is the main substrate for adrenal medulla hormone synthesis
    B. Conversion of pregnenolone to progesterone is the major site of ACTH action
    C. Plasma lipoproteins are major source of cholesterol to adrenals
    D. The foetal adrenal gland are smaller than the adult glands
    E. Zona glomerulosa is the only layer containing 17α-hydroxylase enzyme

4. The hypothalamic–pituitary–adrenal axis plays a key part in maintaining the body's homeostasis, metabolism, and energy consumption. There is an increased production of cortisol when faced with stressors that, in turn, leads to the regulation of multiple functions essential for maintaining homeostasis and cellular integrity.

    Which one of the following physiological changes is attributed to stress-related activation of hypothalamic–pituitary–adrenal axis leading to an enhanced cortisol production?

    A. Decreased free T4 levels
    B. Decreased glycogenolysis
    C. Decreased GnRH
    D. Increased appetite
    E. Increased GH levels

5. The adrenal steroid hormones are derived from cholesterol with plasma lipoproteins acting as the main source for it. The conversion of cholesterol to pregnenolone is one of the key steps in adrenal steroid hormone synthesis.

    Which one of the following enzymes mediates the conversion of cholesterol to pregnenolone in adrenal mitochondria?

    A. 17α-hydroxylase
    B. 11β-hydroxylase
    C. 3β-hydroxyl steroid dehydrogenase (3β-HSD)
    D. 21-hydroxylase
    E. P450 side chain cleavage enzyme (P450 scc)

6. Conversion of 17-hydroxy progesterone to 11 deoxycortisol is the penultimate step in synthesis of adrenal glucocorticoids.

    Which one of the following enzyme mediates conversion of 17-hydroxy progesterone to 11 deoxycortisol?

    A. 17α-hydroxylase
    B. 11β-hydroxylase
    C. 3β-hydroxyl steroid dehydrogenase (3β—HSD)
    D. 21-hydroxylase
    E. P450 side chain cleavage enzyme (P450 scc)

7. The catecholamines (adrenaline and noradrenaline) are synthesized from tyrosine, which is either derived from food or synthesized from phenylalanine in the liver.

   Which one of the following enzyme catalyses the rate-limiting step in catecholamine synthesis?

   A. Catechol-O-methyl transferase
   B. Dopa decarboxylase
   C. Dopamine β-hyroxylase
   D. Monoamine oxidase
   E. Tyrosine kinase

8. Conversion of noradrenaline to adrenaline is mediated by 4-phenyethanolamine-N-methyltransferase (PNMT) enzyme. PNMT is present in the adrenal medulla, lungs, red blood cells, pancreas, and kidneys.

   Which one of the following correctly describes the catecholamine content of the adrenal medulla?

   A. Adrenaline <1% and noradrenaline 99%
   B. Adrenaline 20% and noradrenaline 80%
   C. Adrenaline 50% and noradrenaline 50%
   D. Adrenaline 80% and noradrenaline 20%
   E. Adrenaline 99% and noradrenaline <1%

9. Aldosterone and 11-deoxycorticosterone exert their salt-retaining action by binding to the mineralocorticoid receptors.

   The mineralocorticoid receptors (MRs) are present in all of the following organs/tissues except?

   A. Adipose tissue
   B. Colon
   C. Heart
   D. Kidneys
   E. Liver

10. Cortisol binds to the mineralocorticoid receptor with the same affinity as aldosterone, and circulates in its free form at a much higher concentration as compared with the latter (aldosterone).

    Which one of the following enzymes plays a key role in the conversion of cortisol to inactive cortisone at the tissue level?

    A. 17α-hydroxylase
    B. 3β-hydroxy steroid dehydrogenase (3β-HSD)
    C. 11β-hydroxy steroid dehydrogenase 2 (11β-HSD2)
    D. 21-hydroxylase
    E. P450 scc

11. **A 33-year-old man was referred to the endocrine clinic due to his uncontrolled blood pressure despite being on three anti-hypertensive medications. He had a family history of high blood pressure and haemorrhagic stroke due to aldosterone-producing adenoma (APA).**

    Which one of the following gene mutations has recently been associated with the development of APA?

    A. *CYP11B1*
    B. *DAX1*
    C. *KCNJ5*
    D. *PRKAR1A*
    E. *StAR*

12. **A 35-year-old man presented to his primary care physician with an elevated blood pressure of 160/100 mmHg despite being on anti-hypertensive medication (bendroflumethazide and amlodipine). He had a strong family history of elevated blood pressure and haemorrhagic strokes. His initial blood test results showed hypokalaemia (K 3.2 mmol/L). The diagnosis of secondary hypertension due to primary hyperaldosteronism (PA) is considered.**

    Which one of the following is a recommended criterion to screen for primary hyperaldosteronism?

    A. Adrenal incidentaloma (in a normotensive patient)
    B. Diuretic-induced hypokalaemia
    C. Family history of cerebrovascular disease
    D. Hypertension in pregnancy
    E. Hypertension not controlled by one antihypertensive

13. **A 44-year-old man presented with resistant and uncontrolled hypertension despite being on three different antihypertensive agents. He had a strong family history of stroke and ischaemic heart disease. A diagnosis of PA is considered and a plasma Aldosterone-to-renin ratio (ARR) was arranged as an initial screening test.**

    Which one of the following medications is associated with a false positive plasma aldosterone–serum renin activity test results?

    A. Amlodipine
    B. β-blockers
    C. Doxazosin
    D. Hydralazine
    E. Lisinopril

14. **A 55-year-old gentleman with severe and resistant hypertension underwent further biochemical evaluation to rule out potentially treatable secondary causes for his high blood pressure.**

    ```
    Investigations:
      random ambulant aldosterone  55 pmol/L (100–850)
      plasma renin activity (PRA)  0.1 pmol/mL/h (0.5–3.5)
    ```

    Which one of the following condition can potentially explain these blood test results?

    A. Apparent mineralocorticoid excess
    B. Congenital adrenal hyperplasia
    C. Conn's syndrome
    D. Cushing's syndrome
    E. Renovascular hypertension

15. **A 32-year-old man was referred to the endocrine clinic in view of his uncontrolled and resistant hypertension, despite being on three anti-hypertensive agents (doxazosin, hydralazine, and verapamil). He had strong family history of essential hypertension.**

    ```
    Investigations:
      Na           135 mmol/L (135–45)
      K            3.2 mmol/L (3.5–5.5)
      urea         8.5 mg/dL (5–9)
      creatinine   90 µmol/L (60–115 L)
    ```

    Which one of the following is the most appropriate next step prior to arranging serum ARRin his case?

    A. Correct hypokalaemia
    B. Salt restriction
    C. Stop doxazosin
    D. Stop hydralazine
    E. Stop verapamil

16. **A 36-year-old man presented to the medical assessment unit with a gradual onset headache and high blood pressure. He had no previous history of any significant medical disease. On examination, his blood pressure was 190/110 mmHg, with no evidence of papilloedema.**

```
Investigations:
  Na                            145 mmol/L (135-45)
  K                             4.6 mmol/L (3.5-5.5)
  urea                          8.0 mg/dL (5-9)
  creatinine                    84 µmol/L (60-115)
  random ambulant aldosterone   1645 pmol/L (100-850)
  PRA                           0.1 pmol/mL/h (0.5-3.5)
  CT abdomen                    1.5-cm left adrenal mass
```

Which one of the following is the most appropriate next step in his further management?

A. Adrenal venous sampling

B. Dexamethasone suppression test

C. Laparoscopic left adrenalectomy

D. Start spironolactone

E. Ultrasound-guided biopsy

17. **A 17-year-old was referred to the endocrine clinic with an elevated and difficult to control blood pressure. He also complained of fatigue and muscle pain. On examination, his blood pressure was 180/104 mmHg with no phenotypic features of Cushing's syndrome.**

```
Investigations:
  Na                            140 mmol/L (135-45)
  K                             2.6 mmol/L (3.5-5.5)
  Mg                            1.1 mmol/L (0.7-1.2)
  urea                          6.8 mg/dL (5-9)
  creatinine                    65 µmol/L (60-115)
  random ambulant aldosterone   84 pmol/L (100-850)
  PRA                           0.2 pmol/mL/h (0.5-3.5)
  deoxycorticosterone (DOC)     Low
```

Which one of the following is the probable diagnosis based on his clinical profile?

A. 17β-hydroxylase deficiency

B. Bartter syndrome

C. Conn's syndrome

D. Gitelman syndrome

E. Liddle's syndrome

18. **A 65-year-old woman was referred to the endocrine clinic for further evaluation of her incidentally-detected hypokalaemia. She had a background history of severe oesophageal ulcers for which she was on omeprazole and carbenoxolone therapy. On examination, she had blood pressure of 190/110 mmHg.**

```
Investigations:
  Na                              136 mmol/L (135-45)
  K                               2.8 mmol/L (3.5-5.5)
  venous HCO3                     32 mEq/L (19-25)
  random ambulant aldosterone    65 pmol/L (100-850)
  PRA                             0.3 pmol/mL/h (0.5-3.5)
  DOC                            Low
```

Which one of the following is the probable diagnosis based on her clinical profile?

A. 11β-hydroxylase deficiency
B. Bartter syndrome
C. Conn's syndrome
D. Gitelman syndrome
E. Pseudohyperaldosteronism

19. **A 16-year-old girl was referred to endocrine clinic with features of primary amenorrhoea and delayed puberty.**

On examination, she had blood pressure of 170/108 mmHg, together with a lack of development of secondary sexual characteristics.

```
Investigations:
  Na                              142 mmol/L (135-45)
  K                               2.7 mmol/L (3.5-5.5)
  venous HCO3                     30 mEq/L (19-25)
  random ambulant aldosterone    84 pmol/L (100-850)
  PRA                             0.1 pmol/mL/h (0.5-3.5)
```

Based on her clinical profile, which one of the following is the most likely enzyme defect?

A. 3 β-hydroxysteroid dehydrogenase
B. 11 β-hydroxysteroid dehydrogenase
C. 11 β hydroxylase
D. 17 α-hydroxylase
E. 21-hydroxylase

20. **A 19-year-old student was incidentally detected to have an elevated blood pressure on routine check-up. She had a strong family history of hypertension and haemorrhagic strokes. On examination, she had blood pressure of 160/96 mmHg with no phenotypic features of Cushing's syndrome.**

```
Investigations:
  Na                             136 mmol/L (135-45)
  K                              3.0 mmol/L (3.5-5.5)
  venous HCO₃                    34 mEq/L (19-25)
  random ambulant aldosterone    1450 pmol/L (100-850)
  PRA                            < 0.1 pmol/mL/h (0.5-3.5)
  CT adrenals                    normal adrenal glands
```

Which one of the following management approach/therapies is the most appropriate for the management of her underlying condition?

A. Amiloride

B. Bilateral adrenalectomy

C. Glucocorticoids

D. Mitotane

E. Spironolactone

21. **A 76-year-old man presented with features of rapidly deteriorating glycaemic control and resistant hypertension. On examination, he had facial plethora, proximal myopathy, and easy bruisability.**

```
Investigations:
  urinary free cortisol  3875 nmol/24 h (<280)
Low dose dexamethasone suppression test:
  cortisol  625 nmol/L (<50)
```

CT of the abdomen showed a 4.2-cm adrenal mass (see Figure 4.1).

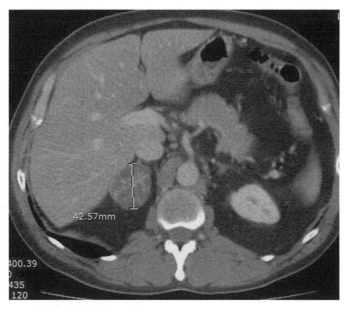

Figure 4.1 CT abdomen transverse view

Reproduced with permission from Dr Nimit Goyal, Consultant Radiologist, Royal Gwent Hospital, Newport, UK

A follow-up scan confirmed liver metastasis. Adrenal biopsy confirmed the diagnosis of adrenocortical tumour.

Which one of the following medications is the preferred treatment option for the management of an inoperable adrenocortical carcinoma?

A. Dexamethasone

B. Ketoconazole

C. Metyrapone

D. Mitotane

E. Octreotide

22. **A 73-year-old man was incidentally detected to have a 3.8-cm right adrenal mass on a non-contrast CT abdomen done to assess his dyspepsia related symptoms.**

    Which of the following radiological features is in keeping with a diagnosis of a likely benign adrenal lesion?

    A. 10 HU density on non-contrast CT
    B. Contrast wash out < 50%
    C. Low lipid content
    D. Non-homogeneous borders
    E. Size 2–4 cm

23. **A 50-year-old man was incidentally detected to have a 2.5-cm left adrenal homogeneous mass with well-defined borders on CT of the abdomen, which was done to evaluate his symptom of dyspepsia. On examination, he had a BMI of 32 kg/m² and blood pressure of 134/70 mmHg. Rest of his general physical and systemic examination was unremarkable.**

    Which one of the following is the most appropriate next step for his further management?

    A. Dexamethasone suppression test (overnight) and urinary metanephrines
    B. MIBG scan
    C. MRI adrenals
    D. Serum ARR
    E. Surgical referral

24. **A 42-year-old woman was incidentally detected to have a 2-cm left adrenal gland mass while she underwent CT of the abdomen to investigate the cause of her pelvic pain and menstrual irregularities.**

    Which one of the following is the most common cause of an incidentally-detected adrenal mass?

    A. Adrenal metastasis
    B. Adrenocortical carcinoma
    C. Conn's syndrome
    D. Non-functional adenoma
    E. Sub-clinical Cushing's disease

25. **A 16-year-old student was incidentally detected to have a 2.8-cm left adrenal gland mass, while she underwent a CT abdomen to rule out acute appendicitis. She had no significant past history of any medical disease. On examination, her blood pressure was 110/70 mmHg, pulse rate of 90 beats/minute with no clinical stigmata of Cushing's disease.**

```
Investigations:
  urinary normetadrenaline  1.5 μmol/24 h (< 4.00)
  urinary metadrenaline     0.3 μmol/24 h (< 2.00)
  9 a.m. cortisol           < 50 nmol/L (after 1 mg overnight
                            dexamethasone)
```

Which one of the following is the most appropriate next step in her further management?

A. Discharge from the clinic

B. MRI adrenals

C. Repeat CT abdomen and biochemistry in 6–12 months

D. Repeat only CT abdomen in 6–12 months

E. Repeat only biochemistry in 6–12 months

26. **A 55-year-old man was incidentally detected to have a 5.5-cm adrenal lesion on CT abdomen done to evaluate symptoms of abdominal pain and weight loss. He had no past history of any significant medical disorder.**

```
Investigations:
  urinary normetadrenaline  0.8 μmol/24 h (< 4.00)
  urinary metadrenaline     0.6 μmol/24 h (< 2.00)
  9 a.m. cortisol           < 50 nmol/L (after 1 mg overnight
                            dexamethasone)
```

Which one of the following is the most appropriate step in his further management?

A. Biopsy

B. Discharge from clinic

C. Laparoscopic FNAC

D. Surgical referral

E. Whole body CT scan

27. A 45-year-old man was incidentally noticed to have a 4.5-cm right adrenal mass with irregular borders and a density of >10 HU on non-contrast CT of the abdomen. On contrast-enhanced CT of the abdomen, there is <20% contrast wash out at 15 minutes. In view of the suspicious radiological features of the mass, the patient was referred to the endocrine surgical team for consideration for an elective adrenalectomy.

    Which one of the following investigations should be arranged prior to an elective adrenalectomy in this patient?

    A. 24-hour urinary fractionated metanephrines
    B. Aldosterone to plasma renin activity ratio
    C. Laparoscopic fine needle aspiration cytology
    D. MIBG scan
    E. PET scan

28. A 22-year-old university student was incidentally detected to have a right adrenal mass on CT of the abdomen, while undergoing evaluation of a possible ectopic pregnancy. She had no past history of any medical disorder. On examination, her blood pressure was 100/60 mmHg with no clinical stigmata of Cushing's disease. Her general physical and systemic examination was unremarkable. She was reported to have a 1.2-cm right adrenal mass with homogeneous appearance and density of –40 HU on non-contrast CT. A further contrast-enhanced CT demonstrated a contrast wash out of >60% at 15 minutes.

    Which one of the following is the most appropriate next step in her management?

    A. Discharge from clinic
    B. MRI adrenal
    C. Repeat CT abdomen in 3–6 months
    D. Serum ARR
    E. Surgical referral

29. A 22-year-old woman presented with recurrent episodes of palpitations, headache, and increased sweating. There were no obvious precipitating factors for these episodes, which could last for 30–40 minutes. On examination, she had elevated blood pressure of 160/94 mmHg with the rest of the general physical and systemic examination being unremarkable. Based on her clinical presentation, a diagnosis of phaeochromocytoma (PH) was considered.

    Which one of the following test is the most sensitive for diagnosis of PH?

    A. 24-hour urinary adrenaline and noradrenaline
    B. 24-hour urinary fractionated metanephrines
    C. 24-hour urinary dopamine
    D. Serum adrenaline and noradrenaline
    E. Serum metanephrines

30. **A 42-year-old woman presented to the accident and emergency department with sudden onset anxiety, palpitations, and headache. On examination, she had blood pressure of 200/120 mmHg, although the fundus examination did not show any papilloedema.**

    ```
    Investigations:
      urinary normetadrenaline  12.8 µmol/24 h (< 4.00)
      urinary metadrenaline     16.0 µmol/24 h (< 2.00)
    ```

    On the basis of her clinical presentation and biochemistry results a diagnosis of intra-adrenal (PH) or extra-adrenal paraganglioma (PGL) was considered.

    Which one of the following investigation is most appropriate for initial localization of the tumour?

    A. CT abdomen
    B. MIBG scan
    C. Octreotide scan
    D. PET scanning
    E. Technetium scan

31. **A 26-year-old woman presented with sudden onset palpitations and anxiety lasting for 30 minutes after taking an over-the-counter medication. On examination, her blood pressure was 170/94 mmHg and she had *cafe au lait* spots on the trunk and lower limbs.**

    Which one of the following characteristics is not suggestive of an underlying diagnosis of PH?

    A. Family history of Von-Hippel–Lindau syndrome
    B. Flushing episodes
    C. Incidental adrenal lesion
    D. Orthostatic hypotension in absence of medication
    E. Paroxysmal hypertension

32. **A 66-year-old woman presented to the medical assessment unit with sudden onset of headache, increased sweating, and palpitations. She had a background medical history of diabetes, hypertension, and osteoarthritis. On examination, she had blood pressure of 140/86 mmHg. Her general physical and systemic examination was unremarkable.**

```
Investigations:
   24-hour urinary adrenaline        1.2 µmol (0-1)
   24-hour urinary metadrenaline     1.4 µmol (< 2.00)
   24-hour urinary noradrenaline     0.4 µmol (0-0.2)
   24-hour urinary normetadrenaline  3.5 µmol (< 4.00)
```

Which one of the following medications is associated with false positive urinary catecholamine results (measured with high pressure liquid chromatography (HPLC))?

A. Acetaminophen

B. Amlodipine

C. Dapagliflozin

D. Diltiazem

E. GLP-1 analogues

33. **A 16-year-old girl presented to medical assessment unit with sudden onset headache, palpitations, and chest tightness. On examination, she had blood pressure of 190/130 mmHg along with tall stature and mucosal neuroma around the mouth.**

```
Investigations:
   24-hour urinary normetadrenaline  6.5 µmol (<4.00)
   24-hour urinary metadrenaline     18.8 µmol (<2.00)
   free T4                           20.2 pmol/L (11.5-22.7)
   TSH                               0.25 mU/L (0.35-5.5)
   corrected calcium                 2.34 mmol/L (2.2-2.6)
   PTH                               4.8 pmol/L (1.6-7.2)
```

Which one of the following gene mutation may be associated with her clinical profile?

A. *MENIN*

B. *NF1*

C. *RET* proto-oncogene

D. *SDHB*

E. *VHL*

34. **A 22-year-old man presented to the accident and emergency department with sudden onset palpitations, increased sweating, and anxiety. He had a background history of a previously removed retinal tumour. He also had a family history of hypertension and haemorrhagic stroke.**

    ```
    Investigations:
      24-hour urinary metadrenaline     2.4 µmol (<2.00)
      24-hour urinary normetadrenaline  16.9 µmol (<4.00)
    ```

    Which one of the following genetic test needs to be arranged based on his clinic profile?

    A. *MENIN*

    B. *NF1*

    C. *RET* proto-oncogene

    D. *SDHB*

    E. *VHL*

35. **A 35-year-old man presented with paroxysmal episodes of sudden onset of palpitations, increased sweating, and anxiety, which became more severe on bending or leaning forward. His general physical and systemic examination was unremarkable, except for elevated blood pressure of 210/96 mmHg, with orthostatic hypotension.**

    ```
    Investigations:
      24-hour urinary normetadrenaline  10.9 µmol (<4.00)
      24-hour urinary metadrenaline     14.0 µmol (<2.00)
      CT of the abdomen                 multiple and bilateral
                                        adrenal masses
    ```

    Which one of the following is <u>not</u> an indication for genetic screening for an individual presenting with clinical features of PH/PGL?

    A. Age <50 years

    B. Bilateral tumours

    C. Malignant tumours

    D. Multiple tumours

    E. Paroxysmal episodes

36. **A 30-year-old teacher was referred to endocrine clinic with paroxysmal symptoms of headache, increased sweating, and anxiety. As she was adopted as a child, no further family history was available. Her general physical and systemic examination was unremarkable.**

    ```
    Investigations:
        24-hour urinary adrenaline         15.2 µmol (0-1)
        24-hour urinary metadrenaline      22.4 µmol (<2.00)
        24-hour urinary noradrenaline      0.5 µmol (0-0.2)
        24-hour urinary normetadrenaline   4.4 µmol (<4.00)
    ```

    Based on her biochemical results, which one of the following genetic test will be most useful in establishing the underlying aetiology?

    A. *MENIN*

    B. *RET* proto-oncogene

    C. *SDHB*

    D. *SDHD*

    E. *VHL*

37. **A 26-year-old woman presented to the clinic with an incidentally-detected painless neck lump. She had a background medical history of eczema and was not on any medications. Her father had undergone removal of a neck lump, which turned out to be benign when he was in his 4th decade.**

    ```
    Investigations:
        24-hour urinary metadrenaline      1.4 µmol (<2.00)
        24-hour urinary normetadrenaline   2.5 µmol (<4.00)
        neck ultrasound                    possible carotid body
                                           tumour
    ```

    Based on the location of the lump and family history a diagnosis of familial PGLs was considered.

    Which one of the following gene mutations is commonly associated with parasympathetic PGLs?

    A. *NFI*

    B. *RET* proto-oncogene

    C. *SDHB*

    D. *SDHD*

    E. *VHL*

38. A 22-year-old woman presented to the endocrine clinic with symptoms of recurrent episodes of palpitations and increased sweating lasting for 5–10 minutes. On examination, her blood pressure was 150/90 mmHg. The general physical and systemic examination was unremarkable.

```
Investigations:
  24-hour urinary metadrenaline     2.5 µmol (<2.00)
  24-hour urinary normetadrenaline  4.9 µmol (<4.00)
  CT of the adrenal gland           normal adrenal glands
```

Which one of the following is the most appropriate next investigation for localization of intra-extra adrenal PGLs?

A. MIBG scan
B. MRI abdomen
C. Octreoscan
D. PET scan
E. Whole body CT scan

39. A 62-year-old woman complained of nasal stuffiness, together with giddiness on standing up, while she is on gradually increasing dose of phenoxybenzamine started 6 days ago to achieve α-blockage prior to an elective adrenalectomy. She had recently been diagnosed with a left-sided PH measuring 3.5 cm on CT of the abdomen. On examination, she had a resting heart rate of 124 beats/minute, with a significant postural drop of 25 mmHg on standing up.

Which one of the following is the most appropriate next step in her further management?

A. Add metoprolol
B. Increase phenoxybenzamine dose
C. Reduce phenoxybenzamine dose
D. Stop phenoxybenzamine
E. Switch to metoprolol

40. **A 55-year-old man presented with symptoms of paroxysmal episodes of palpitations, headache, and elevated blood pressure. He had no family history of sudden cardiac death or multiple endocrine neoplasia. On examination, he had an elevated blood pressure of 180/104 mmHg with no stigmata of neurofibromatosis.**

```
Investigations:
    24-hour urinary metadrenaline     22.4 µmol (<2.00)
    24-hour urinary normetadrenaline  4.5 µmol (<4.00)
    CT of the adrenal gland           3-cm left-sided adrenal
                                      tumour
```

Which one of the following is the most appropriate next step in his further management?

A. Elective adrenalectomy

B. Genetic screening

C. MIBG scan

D. PET scan

E. Radiotherapy

41. **A 26-year-old man was admitted to the medical assessment unit with progressive lethargy and malaise for the previous 6 weeks. He was previously well and played football for a local club. For the last few weeks he had felt exhausted after playing for 10–15 minutes. He had a family history of Type 1 DM and autoimmune hypothyroidism. On examination, he had pigmentation of the palmer surface of the hand and buccal mucosa, with the rest of his general physical and systemic examination being unremarkable.**

```
Investigations:
    Na         130 mmol/L (135-145)
    K          5.9 mg/dL (3.5-5.5)
    urea       10.5 mg/dL (5-9)
    creatinine 95 µmol/L (60-115)
    calcium    2.65 mmol/L (2.2-2.6)
    phosphate  0.94 mmol/L (0.8-1.5)
```

Antibodies directed against which one of the following enzymes have been linked with his underlying clinical condition?

A. 3β-HSD

B. 11β-hydroxylase

C. 17α-hydroxylase

D. 17, 20 lyase

E. 21-hyroxylase

42. **A 46-year-old man was referred to the endocrinology team for further assessment of his symptoms of fatigue, malaise, and weight loss. He had a background history of cirrhosis, with portal hypertension due to alcoholic liver disease. On examination, he looked cachectic and had peripheral stigmata of liver failure.**

```
Investigations:
  albumin                            18 g/L (30—50)
  alkaline phosphatase (ALP)         275 U/L (50-125)
  alanine transaminase (ALT)         142 mU/L (05-58)
  bilirubin                          2.1 nmol/L (0.1-1)
  0 hour cortisol                    155 nmol/L
  30 minutes cortisol (post-ACTH)    396 nmol/L (>500)
```

Which one of the following is the most appropriate next step in his further management?

A. Measure 21 α-hydroxylase antibodies
B. Measure salivary cortisol after ACTH
C. Repeat short synacthen test in 1 week
D. Start hydrocortisone
E. Start hydrocortisone and fludrocortsione

43. **An 18-year-old man presented with symptoms of progressive weight loss and malaise over a period of last 4 months. He had background history of cerebellar ataxia and in-coordination, for which he was under neurology clinic follow-up. On examination, he had features of gait disturbance and emotional lability.**

```
Investigations:
  Na                     131 mmol/L (135-145)
  K                      5.8 mmol/L (3.5-5.5)
  urea                   10.5 mg/dL (5-9)
  creatinine             95 µmol/L (60-115)
  calcium                2.65 mmol/L (2.2-2.6)
  0 hour cortisol        44 nmol/L
  30 minutes post-ACTH   128 nmol/L (>500)
```

Which one of the following investigations will be useful in establishing the underlying diagnosis in his clinical context?

A. 17α-hydroxylase antibodies
B. 21-hyroxylase antibodies
C. Adrenal biopsy
D. MRI brainstem
E. Very long chain fatty acids (VLCFA)

44. **A 48-year-old woman presented to her GP with symptoms of progressive weight gain, fatigue, and menstrual irregularity. On examination, she had facial plethora, central obesity, increased facial and body hair, proximal myopathy, and easy bruisability. Based on her signs and symptoms, a clinical suspicion of Cushing's syndrome was raised and a 24-hour urinary free cortisol measurement is arranged.**

    Which one of the following clinical features is relatively discriminatory for the diagnosis of Cushing's syndrome?

    A. Facial plethora
    B. Hirsutism
    C. Stretch marks
    D. Weight gain
    E. Worsening glycaemic control

45. **A 50-year-old man presented to the clinic with progressive weight gain and easy bruisability. He had a background medical history of epilepsy and type 2 diabetes, and he was taking phenytoin and metformin tablets. On examination, he had central obesity, facial fullness, and thin skin, although there was no evidence of proximal myopathy or facial plethora.**

    Which one of the following test is most appropriate for initial screening of Cushing's syndrome in his clinical scenario?

    A. 24-hour urinary free cortisol
    B. Insulin tolerance test
    C. Low dose dexamethasone suppression test
    D. Overnight dexamethasone suppression test
    E. Plasma ACTH levels

46. **A 24-year-old woman presented to her GP with symptoms of weight gain, excessive facial hair growth, and menstrual irregularities. She was on metformin and oral contraceptive pills for a suspected diagnosis of polycystic ovarian syndrome. On examination, she had increased BMI, hirsutism, facial puffiness, and lower abdominal stria. Based on her symptoms and signs, a clinical suspicion of Cushing's syndrome was raised.**

    Which one of the following investigations will be most appropriate for initial screening of Cushing's syndrome in her clinical scenario?

    A. 24-hour urinary free cortisol
    B. CT adrenals
    C. Insulin tolerance test
    D. Overnight dexamethasone suppression test
    E. Plasma ACTH levels

47. **A 44-year-old woman presented to the clinic with progressive weight gain, lethargy, and easy bruisability. She had background medical history of type 2 diabetes and hypertension. On examination, she had central obesity, lower abdominal striae, and proximal myopathy. Based on a clinical suspicion of Cushing' syndrome, a mid-night salivary cortisol measurement is arranged as an initial screening test.**

   Which one of the following may be associated with a false positive salivary cortisol test result?

   A. Anti-epileptic medications
   B. Chewing tobacco
   C. Hepatic failure
   D. Oral contraceptive pills
   E. Renal failure

48. **A 26-year-old woman presented with facial puffiness and easy bruisability, while she was in her first trimester of pregnancy. On examination, she had facial plethora, lower abdominal purple stria, and proximal myopathy. A clinical suspicion of Cushing's syndrome was raised based on her signs and symptoms.**

   Which one of the following is the most appropriate screening test for the diagnosis of Cushing' s syndrome in pregnancy?

   A. 24-hour urinary free cortisol
   B. CT adrenals
   C. Insulin tolerance test
   D. Overnight dexamethasone suppression test
   E. Salivary cortisol

49. **A 22-year-old man was referred to endocrine clinic with features of easy bruisability and a recent fragility fracture. He denied the use of any illicit drugs or excess alcohol consumption. He had no previous medical history of any chronic illness, weight loss, or steroid use. On examination, he had buccal and perioral lentigenes, facial plethora, proximal myopathy, and lower abdominal stria.**

   ```
   Investigations:
     24-hour urinary free cortisol   elevated ×3 times normal limit
     mid-night salivary cortisol     raised
     ECHO                            atrial myxoma
   ```

   All of the following are known endocrine manifestations of his underlying syndrome except?

   A. Adrenocortical rests
   B. GH secreting tumour
   C. Leydig-cell tumour
   D. Multiple thyroid nodules
   E. Primary hyperaldosteronism

50. A 24-year-old Hispanic woman was referred to the endocrine clinic with symptoms of menstrual irregularity and excessive facial hair growth. On examination she had a BMI of 22 kg/m² and features of hirsutism.

Investigations:
```
FSH                      2.8 U/L (follicular 0.5-5, mid-cycle
                         8-33, luteal 2-8)
LH                       8.0 U/L (follicular 3-12, mid-cycle
                         20-80, luteal 3-16)
oestradiol               74 pmol/L (follicular 17-260, luteal
                         180-1100)
andrestendione           22 nmol/L (4-10.2)
17- OH progesterone  13 nmol/L (follicular <5)
```

Which one of the following investigations is the most appropriate to establish the underlying diagnosis in her case?

A. Aldosterone to plasma renin activity
B. CT adrenals
C. Short synacthen test (measuring 17- hydroxy progesterone, 17-OHP)
D. Testosterone levels
E. Ultrasound pelvis

51. A 20-year-old man was reviewed in endocrine clinic on a routine follow up visit. He had background history of classic—congenital adrenal hyperplasia (CAH) diagnosed at birth and has been on life-long prednisolone (7.5 mg/day) and fludrocortisone (100 μg/day) replacement therapy. On examination, he had no phenotypic features of Cushing's syndrome. There was no palpable testicular lump on genital examination.

Investigations:
```
androstenedione          26.5 nmol/L (4.4-10.6)
17-OHP                   20.0 nmol/L (< 3)
plasma renin activity  4.5 pmol/mL/h (1.1-2.7)
```

Which one of the following is the most appropriate next step in his management?

A. Check compliance
B. CT abdomen
C. Increase prednisolone dose
D. Increase prednisolone, as well as fludrocortisone dose
E. Switch to dexamethasone

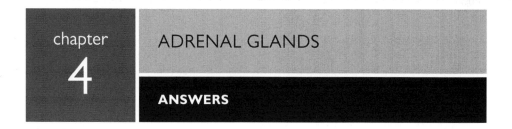

1. B. The adrenal glands weigh around 4–5 g and are located retroperitoneally near the upper pole of the kidneys. These are made up of two embryologically distinct layers—the outer cortex, which is mesodermal in origin, and the inner medulla, derived from neuroectoderm. The adrenal cortex in turn is composed of three different layers:

- Zona glomerulosa.
- Zona fasciculate.
- Zona reticularis.

The zona glomerulosa secrets aldosterone, the zona fasciculata is involved primarily in glucocorticoid synthesis, and the zona reticularis is the site of androgen (dihydroepiandrostenedione, androstenedione) and, to a smaller extent, glucocorticoids synthesis.

Greenspan F and Gardner D. Basic and clinical endocrinology. McGraw-Hill Medical, 2011.

2. B. The secretion of mineralocorticoids from zona glomerulosa is regulated primarily by angiotensin 2, serum potassium levels and ACTH. Atrial natriureitc peptide and dopamine can also influence the secretion of mineralocorticoids.

ACTH plays a key part in regulation of glucocorticoids secretion from zona fasciculata. Cytokines such as interleukin-1, interleukin-6, and TNFα along with catecholamines also have a minor role in the regulation of glucocorticoid secretion by zona fasciculata.

Nussey S and Whitehead S. Endocrinology, An integrated approach. Bios Scientific publishers, 2001.

3. C. At about 4 months gestation, the adrenal glands are about four times the size of the kidneys, although there is a significant regression of the adrenal cortex at birth. The zona fasciculata starts to develop from age of 4–5 years in children.

Plasma lipoproteins are the major source of cholesterol to the adrenal glands. The conversion of cholesterol to pregnenolone is the major site of action of ACTH. The zona glomerulosa is deficient in 17α-hydroxylase and, as a result, it cannot produce cortisol or androgens.

The zona reticularis continues to develop till age 20–25 years, with adrenal androgens playing a role in the development of pubic and axillary hair. This layer undergoes regression after the reproductive phase of life. The adrenal androgens do not play any significant role in adult males, although in adult females they are the main source of androgens. Excess adrenal androgen production in women may result in menstrual irregularities, acne, and features of hirsutism. The adrenal androgens are secreted in increasing amounts at age 6–7 years in girls and 7–8 years age in boys. The axillary and pubic hair regions are the most sensitive androgen-dependent areas.

Greenspan F and Gardner D. Basic and Clinical Endocrinology. McGraw-Hill Medical, 2011.

4. C. The stress-mediated response to increased cortisol production as a result of activation of hypothalamic–pituitary–adrenal (HPA) axis includes CRH-induced anorexia, GnRH, and GH suppression. The stress-induced increased levels of endogenous glucocorticoids result in increased glycogenolysis, hepatic gluconeogenesis, and increased LDL cholesterol levels.

TSH secretion, as well as peripheral conversion of FT4 to biologically active FT3 is reduced by stress-mediated activation of the HPA axis, although the FT4 levels remain within the normal limit.

O'Connor T, O'Halloran DJ, Shanahan F. The stress response and the hypothalamic-pituitary-adrenal axis: from molecule to melancholia. Quarterly Journal of Medicine 2000; 93(6): 323–333.

5. E. The free cholesterol transfer from the outer to inner mitochondrial membrane is facilitated by steroid acute regulatory protein (see Figure 4.2). This is followed by side chain cleavage of cholesterol, mediated by P450 scc enzyme leading to the formation of pregnenolone. The conversion of pregnenolone to 17-hyroxy pregnenolone is regulated by 17α-hydroxylase enzyme. 3β-hydroxyl steroid dehydrogenase enzyme mediates conversion of 17α-pregnenolone to 17α-progesterone. 21-hydroxylase mediates conversion of 17α-progesterone to 11-deoxycortisol, while 11β-hydroxylase leads to conversion of 11-deoxycortisol to cortisol.

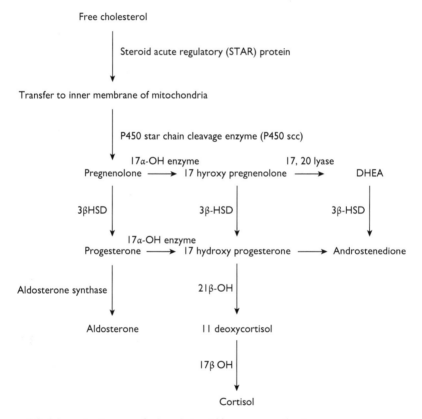

Figure 4.2 Schematic diagram of adrenal steroid hormone synthesis

Greenspan F and Gardner D. Basic and clinical endocrinology. McGraw-Hill Medical, 2011.

6. D. Enzyme 21-hydroxylase mediates the conversion of 17-hydroxy progesterone to 11-deoxycortisol. The autoimmune adrenal insufficiency is characterized by elevated auto-antibodies to 21-hydroxylase enzyme leading to reduced/absent cortisol synthesis in adrenals.

Nussey S and Whitehead S. Endocrinology, An integrated approach. Bios Scientific publishers, 2001.

7. E. Tyrosine kinase catalyses the rate-limiting step in catecholamine synthesis (conversion of tyrosine to dopa). Dopamine to noradrenaline conversion is mediated by enzyme dopamine β-hyroxylase. Monoamine oxidase regulates the catecholamine content of the neurons by inactivating the excess intracellular noradrenaline.

In PHs, catechol-O-methyl transferase mediates the conversion of adrenaline and noradrenaline to the metabolically-inactive compounds metadrenaline and metnoradrenaline, respectively, which are released into the circulation and excreted in urine.

Melmed S, Polonsky K, Larsen P, and Kronenberg H. Williams textbook of endocrinology (12th edn). Saunders Publishers, 2012.

8. D. The normal human adrenal medulla has about 80% adrenaline and 20% noradrenaline. The conversion of noradrenaline to adrenaline is mediated by PNMT enzyme, which is induced by the high concentration of cortisol present in the adrenal medulla (due to venous blood flow from the adjacent adrenal medulla). Non-adrenal tissues contribute only minimally to circulating adrenaline. In contrast to normal adrenal medulla, PH cells usually contain more noradrenaline compared with adrenaline, especially the extra-adrenal PGLs.

9. E. The MR are present in adipose tissue, colon, kidneys, cardiomyocytes, sweat glands, vascular endothelium, and pituitary gland. Aldosterone and 11-DOC have an equal affinity to bind to MR, although the former (aldosterone) is quantitatively a more important mineralocorticoid hormone as 30–50% of it circulates in an unbound form compared with the later DOC, which is >95% bound by the cortisol-binding globulin.

Melmed S, Polonsky K, Larsen P, and Kronenberg H. Williams textbook of endocrinology (12th edn). Saunders Publishers, 2012.

10. C. The conversion of cortisol to inactive cortisone at the tissue level is mediated by enzyme 11β-hydroxy steroid dehydrogenase type 2 (11β-HSD2), which protects the MR from excessive cortisol binding. Glycyrrhizic acid (the active ingredient of liquorice) inhibits 11β-HSD2 leading to increased free cortisol being available to bind to the MR, resulting in hypertension and hypokalaemia. Another enzyme, 11β-HSD type 1 (11β-HSD1), present in skin and liver, mediates the conversion of cortisone to cortisol.

11. C. Glomerular specific K channel gene (*KCNJ5*) has been linked with the development of aldosterone-producing adenoma. *CYP11B1* gene mutation is associated with the development of the atypical variant of congenital adrenal hyperplasia (CAH). *DAX1* mutation is associated with the development of X-linked adrenal hypoplasia congenital. Steroidogenic acute regulatory protein (*StAR*) gene mutation has been linked with the development of congenital lipoid adrenal hyperplasia. A mutation in *PRKAR1A* gene has been associated with the development of primary pigmented nodular adrenocortical disease (PPNAD).

Boulkroun S, Beuschlein F, Rossi G, et al. Prevalence, clinical, and molecular correlates of KCNJ5 mutations in primary aldosteronism. Hypertension, 2012; 59: 592–598.

12. B. The recommended criteria for screening for PA in patients with hypertension include:
1. Young age.
2. Diuretic-induced or spontaneous hypokalaemia.
3. Resistant hypertension (to more than two anti-hypertensive medications).
4. Severe hypertension (systolic >160 mmHg, diastolic >100 mmHg).
5. Adrenal incidentaloma (1% of patients may have PA).
6. A strong family history of early onset hypertension or haemorrhagic strokes at a young age.
7. Metabolic alkalosis.

PA was first described by J. W. Conn in 1954. It has the following seven subtypes:

- APA
- Bilateral idiopathic hyperaldosteronism (IHA)
- Unilateral hyperplasia
- Familial hyperaldosteronism
- Glucocorticoid remedial hyperaldosteronism
- Aldosterone producing adrenal carcinoma
- Ectopic aldosterone producing carcinoma

Funder J, Carey R, Fardella C et al. Case Detection, Diagnosis, and Treatment of Patients with Primary Hyperaldosteronism: An Endocrine Society Clinical Practice Guideline. Journal of Clinical Endocrinology & Metabolism, 93: 3266–81, 2008.

13. B. Anti-hypertensive agents and other medications can influence the results of serum ARR activity ratio test results as shown in Table 4.1.

Table 4.1 Effect of various medications on serum ARR

False positive	False negative	No impact on results
β blockers	ACE inhibitors	Doxazosin
Clonidine	Angiotensin receptor blockers	Hydralazine
Hormone replacement therapy	Bendroflumethazide	Terazosin
Methyldopa	Calcium channel blockers	Verapamil
NSAIDs	Eplerenone	
Oral contraceptive pills	Spironolactone	

Funder J, Carey R, Fardella C et al. Case Detection, Diagnosis, and Treatment of Patients with Primary Hyperaldosteronism: An Endocrine Society Clinical Practice Guideline. Journal of Clinical Endocrinology & Metabolism, 93: 3266–81, 2008.

Turner H and Wass J. Oxford handbook of endocrinology and diabetes. Oxford University Press.

14. D. Aldosterone levels vary with age, time of the day, salt intake and renal function. The measurement of serum aldosterone should be done as an ambulatory test (8–10 a.m.) with patient having an unrestricted salt intake (caution required in patients with uncontrolled hypertension) and hypokalaemia needs to be corrected prior to the test.

The serum aldosterone to plasma rennin activity ratio result may provide clue to an alternate aetiology for elevated hypertension as shown in Table 4.2.

Table 4.2 Aldosterone and plasma renin activity in various conditions causing secondary hypertension

Condition	Aldosterone	Plasma renin activity
Primary hyperaldosteronism	high	low
Renovascular hypertension	high	high
Cushing's syndrome	low	low

Wass J, Stewart P, Amiel S, and Davies M. Oxford textbook of Endocrinology & Diabetes (2nd edition, July 2011). Oxford University Press. ISBN 9780199235292.

15. A. Hypokalaemia needs to be corrected prior to the measurement of serum ARR. Verapamil, Hydralazine, Doxazosin do not effect serum ARR.

False positive test can be seen with β blocker, methyldopa, clonidine and non-steroidal anti-inflammatory agents (NSAIDs). These agents need to be stopped for 2 weeks prior to the measurement of serum ARR. False positive test seen if patient is on oral contraceptive pills (OCP) or hormone replacement therapy (HRT) as oestrogen containing medications lower the direct renin concentration (no effect on plasma renin activity).

Spironolactone and eplerenone use can lead to false negative serum ARRtest results as a result these agents need to be stopped at least 4–6 weeks prior to the test. False negative test results can be seen if patient is on bendroflumethazide, ACE inhibitors and calcium channel blockers (dihydro-pyridine group, e.g. amlodipine, nifedipine).

16. A. Adrenal CT has several limitations including inability to detect small aldosterone producing adenomas (APAs) or these lesions getting incorrectly labelled as bilateral idiopathic hyperaldos-teronism (IHA). The apparent adrenal nodules on CT may actually represent an area of hyperpla-sia. Incidentally-detected adrenal lesions are also indistinguishable from APAs on CT. In view of the above-mentioned limitations of radiological imaging studies, it is recommended that adrenal venous sampling should be arranged for patients with a possible APA, if surgery is deemed practical. See Figure 4.3.

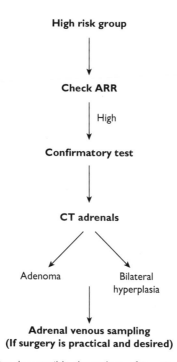

Figure 4.3 Flow chart depicting the possible chronology of investigations for a suspected patient with primary hyperaldosteronism; ARR = aldosterone to renin ratio

Funder J, Carey R, Fardella C, et al. Case detection, diagnosis, and treatment of patients with primary hyperaldosteronism: an Endocrine Society clinical practice guideline. Journal of Clinical Endocrinology & Metabolism 2008; 93: 3266–3281.

Wass J, Stewart P, Amiel S, and Davies M. Oxford textbook of endocrinology & diabetes (2nd edn). Oxford University Press, 2011.

17. E. Liddle's syndrome is an autosomal dominant condition due to a mutation in the *SCNN1B* or *SCNN1G* gene (representing epithelial sodium channels) leading to enhanced Na reabsorption from renal tubules. Patients may present at an early age with high blood pressure, hypokalaemia, metabolic alkalosis in the presence of suppressed serum aldosterone, plasma renin activity, and low/unmeasurable DOC levels. The treatment includes a low-salt diet, with potassium sparing diuretics, such as amiloride and triamterene. See Table 4.3.

Table 4.3 Clinical and biochemical characteristics of various conditions leading to hypokalaemia

Condition	Characteristic features	Blood pressure	Potassium	Aldosterone	Renin
Conn's syndrome	Uncontrolled and resistant hypertension	High	Low/normal	High	Low
Atypical variants of CAH 17α-hydroxylase deficiency	Lack of synthesis of androgens and/or oestrogens. Increase DOC, 18-OH corticosterone	High	Low/normal	Low	Low
11β-hydroxylase deficiency	Increased plasma androgens, 11 deoxycortisol, urinary 17-ketosteroids	High	Low/normal	Low	Low
Apparent cortisol excess	11β-HSD2 deficiency Low DOC	High	Low/normal	Low	Low
Liddle's syndrome	Enhanced renal tubular Na reabsorption	High	Low/normal	Low	Low
Bartter syndrome	Renal tubular defect	Normal	Low	High	High
Gitelman syndrome	Low Mg/Low calcium Renal tubular defect (mutation in the *SCL12A3* gene)	Normal	Low	High	High

Turner H and Wass J. Oxford handbook of endocrinology and diabetes. Oxford University Press, 2009.

18. E. Pseudohyperaldosteronism is characterized by clinical features (hypertension, hypokalaemia, and metabolic alkalosis) consistent with excessive mineralocorticoid secretion in the presence of low or suppressed aldosterone/DOC levels. It may be seen in the presence of 11β-hydroxysteroid dehydrogenase type 2 (11β-HSD2) enzyme deficiency (due to a genetic mutation), which mediates the conversion of cortisol to inactive cortisone at the tissue level.

Ingestion of liquorice or carbenoxolone (a synthetic derivative of glycyrrhetinic acid) can inhibit 11β-HSD2 enzyme, leading to excessive availability of cortisol to bind to MR, inducing features of pseudohyperaldosteronism. The diagnosis can be confirmed by measurement of the urinary tetrahydrocortisol to tetrahydrocortisone ratio (increased urinary tetrahydrocortisol to tetrahydrocortisone ratio).

Sonita B, Mooney J, Gaudet L, and Touyz R. Pseudohyperaldosteronism, liquorice and hypertension. Journal of Clinical Hypertension (Greenwich), 2008; 10 (2): 153–157.

19. D. Aldosterone and DOC are endogenous mineralocorticoid hormones secreted by zona glomerulosa and fasciculate, respectively. Aldosterone has low affinity to bind with corticosteroid-binding globulin (CBG) and mainly circulates in free form, making it biologically more relevant as a mineralocorticoid hormone (compared with DOC, which binds more avidly to CBG).

17 α-hydroxylase deficiency syndrome is characterized by presence of hypertension, hypokalaemia and low aldosterone as well as low plasma renin activity along with an elevated non-17 α-hydroxylated steroid levels. Females with this enzyme defect have primary amenorrhoea with sexual infantilism, while men may have features of pseudohermaphroditism. Treatment is with glucocorticoids to suppress ACTH secretion, while female patients may, in addition, require oestrogen replacement therapy.

Costa-Santos M, Kater CE, Auchus RJ, et al. Brazilian Congenital Adrenal Hyperplasia Multicenter Study Group. Two prevalent CYP17 mutations and genotype-phenotype correlations in 24 Brazilian patients with 17-hydroxylase deficiency. Journal of Clinical Endocrinology & Metabolism 2004; 89(1): 49–60.

Krone N and Arlt W. Genetics of congenital adrenal hyperplasia. Best Practice Research in Clinical Endocrinology & Metabolism, 2009; 23(2): 181–192.

20. C. Glucocorticoid remedial hyperaldosteronism (GRA) is an autosomal dominant disorder characterized by the presence of a chimeric gene, which leads to fusion of the regulatory region of 11β-hydroxylase gene to the coding sequence of aldosterone synthase. As a result, patients have an ACTH-induced increased synthesis of aldosterone, 18-hydroxycortisol, and 18-oxocortisol, and may present with features of mineralocorticoid excess (hypertension, hypokalaemia, and metabolic alkalosis). A family history of primary aldosteronism and/or haemorrhagic strokes should prompt a clinician to explore the possible presence of GRA. Treatment is with a low dose of dexamethasone to suppress ACTH activity. Genetic analysis is usually required to confirm the diagnosis.

Halperin F and Dluhy R. Glucocorticoid remedial hyperaldosteronism. Endocrinology Metabolism Clinics of North America, 2011; 40(2): 333–341.

21. D. Mitotane is the preferred medication used for the management of inoperable adreno-cortical carcinoma. It is an adrenolytic drug that inhibits several enzymes involved in steroid/mineralocorticoid synthesis, including side chain cleavage, 11β-hydroxylase and 3β-hydroxy steroid hydrogenase (3β-HSD). It controls the cortisol hypersecretion-related symptoms in 70–75% of patients, although it is associated with the development of frequent and serious side effects, including nausea, vomiting, hypogonadism, thyroid dysfunction, neurotoxicity, and adrenocortical suppression, which may warrant glucocorticoid replacement and close monitoring.

Schteingart D, Doherty G, Gauger P, et al. Management of patients with adrenal carcinoma: recommendations of an international consensus conference. Endocrine-Related Cancer, 2005; 12: 667–680.

22. E. The following radiological features are in keeping with a benign adrenal lesion:

- <10 Hounsfield units (HU) on non-contrast CT (e.g. myelolipomas <–30 HU).
- Contrast wash out >50% in 15 minutes.
- High lipid content.
- Homogeneous borders.

Nieman LK. Approach to the patient with an adrenal incidentaloma. Journal of Clinical Endocrinology & Metabolism, 2010; 95(9): 4106–4113.

Zeiger M, Thompson G, Duh Q, et al. American Association of Clinical Endocrinologists and American Association of Endocrine Surgeons. Medical Guidelines for the Management of Adrenal Incidentalomas. Endocrine Practice, 2009; 15(Suppl. 1)–20.

23. A. The prevalence of adrenal incidentaloma has been reported to be about 8–9% and 2–6%, based on various autopsy and radiological series, respectively. There has been a significant increase in the detection of adrenal incidentalomas with the advent of newer and more sophisticated radiological investigations. Any patient with adrenal incidentaloma measuring <4 cm with benign radiological features (homogeneous mass, well-defined borders and <10 HU on non-contrast CT) should undergo clinical and biochemical evaluation to assess the functional status of the lesion. The incidence of sub-clinical Cushing's disease and PH in adrenal lesions has been reported as being between 3 and 5%, based on data from various retrospective studies. All patients should have urinary/serum metanephrine measurement to exclude PH, and overnight dexamethasone suppression test or midnight salivary cortisol measurement is the preferred screening test to rule out Cushing's disease. Conn's syndrome needs to be excluded only if the patient has hypertension.

24. D. Table 4.4 shows a list of various functional or non-functional lesions presenting as an adrenal incidentaloma

Table 4.4 Causes of adrenal incidental masses

Non-functional (85–90%)	Functional (10–15%)
Adenoma	Aldosterone secreting
Carcinoma	Catecholamine secreting
Cyst	Cortisol secreting
Haemorrhage	
Myelolipoma	

25. C. All patients with non-functional adrenal incidentaloma >1 cm in size should have repeat clinical, biochemical, and radiological reassessment at an interval of 6 months to 1 year. If the repeat radiology does not show any change in size of the lesion, with no clinical and/or biochemical features of hormone excess, most European centres do not advocate further follow-up routinely.

According to the American Association of Clinical Endocrinologists (AACE) and American Association of Endocrine Surgeons (AAES) guidelines, adrenal masses that appear to be benign should be reimaged at 3–6 months, then annually for 1–2 years. Functional status of the lesion needs to be assessed on a yearly basis for 5 years. Any lesion that grows by >1 cm or shows functional overactivity needs to be removed by adrenalectomy.

Nieman LK. Approach to the patient with an adrenal incidentaloma. Journal of Clinical Endocrinology & Metabolism, 2010; 95(9): 4106–4113.

Zeiger M, Thompson G, Duh Q, et al. American Association of Clinical Endocrinologists and American Association of Endocrine Surgeons. Medical Guidelines for the Management of Adrenal Incidentalomas. Endocrine Practice, 2009; 15(Suppl 1): 1–20.

26. D. The size of adrenal lesion correlates with increased risk of developing malignancy. Adrenal masses measuring >4, but >6 cm have, respectively, 6 and 25% likelihood of being malignant. The following features are associated with an increased risk of malignancy in an incidentally-detected adrenal lesion:

- Size >4 cm.
- Irregular and non-homogeneous margins.
- Non-contrast CT density >10 HU.
- Wash-out of contrast (after 15 minutes) <40%.

Nieman LK. Approach to the patient with an adrenal incidentaloma. Journal of Clinical Endocrinology & Metabolism, 2010; 95(9): 4106–4113.

Zeiger M, Thompson G, Duh Q, et al. American Association of Clinical Endocrinologists and American Association of Endocrine Surgeons. Medical Guidelines for the Management of Adrenal Incidentalomas. Endocrine Practice, 2009; 15(Suppl 1): 1–20.

27. A. About 5% of the patients with adrenal incidentalomas have been reported to have PHs as an underlying diagnosis. The radiological appearance of a PH may include a large tumour, areas of haemorrhage, and necrosis with irregular borders, which may mimic an adrenal carcinoma. As a result, all patients with suspicions radiological features of an adrenal carcinoma should have 24-hour fractionated urinary metanephrine and/or serum metanephrine measurement to exclude the diagnosis of PH.

Barzon L, Sonino N, Fallo F, et al. Prevalence and natural history of adrenal incidentalomas. European Journal of Endocrinology, 2003; 149: 273–285.

Grumbach M, Biller B, Braunstein G, et al. NIH state-of-the-science statement on management of the clinically inapparent adrenal mass ('incidentaloma'). NIH Consens State Sci Statements. 2002; 19: 1–25.

Young W. The incidentally discovered adrenal mass. New England Journal of Medicine, 2007; 356: 601–610.

28. A. The radiological features in this patient are consistent with a myelolipoma; functional status of such lesions is only evaluated if it is clinically indicated. This patient can be discharged from the clinic without the need for repeat radiological investigation

Kapoor A, Morris T, and Rebello R. Guidelines for the management of the incidentally discovered adrenal mass. Canadian Urology Assocociation Journal, 2011; 5 (4): 241–247.

Vassilatou E, Vryonidou A, Michalopoulou S, et al. Hormonal activity of adrenal incidentalomas: results from a long-term follow-up study. Clinical Endocrinology (Oxford), 2009; 70: 674–679.

29. E. According to WHO definition (2004), the PGLs can be divided into two main categories: intra-adrenal (also historically known as PH) or extra-adrenal. The extra-adrenal PGLs are, in turn, divided into sympathetic or parasympathetic, based on their chain of origin. Intra-adrenal (PH) and extra-adrenal sympathetic PGLs are characterized by increased secretion of adrenaline and noradrenaline. The catecholamine release from these tumours may occur intermittently or at a low rate, which may lead to a false negative result on urinary measurement of these hormones.

The catecholamines are metabolized to metadrenaline and normetadrenaline (also known as metanephrines) in chromaffin cells. The conversion to metanephrines occurs within the tumour, independent of catecholamine release. Therefore, metanephrine measurement is more sensitive, as well as specific than catecholamine measurement for the diagnosis of PH and PGL, although it is yet to be used widely due to limited availability and high costs.

The sensitivity and specificity of biochemical tests used for the diagnosis of PH and PGL is shown in Table 4.5.

Table 4.5 Sensitivity and specificity of biochemical tests used for diagnosis of PH and PGL

Test	Sensitivity (%)	Specificity (%)
24-hour urinary adrenaline and noradrenaline	85	88
24-hour urinary metanephrines	97	70
Serum adrenaline and noradrenaline	84	80
Serum metanephrines	99	89

Chen H, Sipple R, O'Dorisio MS, et al. The North American Neuroendocrine Tumor Society Consensus Guideline for the Diagnosis and Management of Neuroendocrine Tumors. Pancreas, 2010; 39: 775–783

30. B. In patients with suspected PH or PGL urinary metanephrine/catecholamines should be measured as a part of initial screening. CT of the abdomen remains the initial modality of choice to localize the tumour if biochemistry results are suggestive of the diagnosis of PH or extra-adrenal PGLs (which are mostly intra-abdominal).

MIBG scanning should be considered for patients suspected with PH or PGL, if the initial CT fails to localize the tumour or to assess for any possible metastasis (e.g. in patients with Von Hippel–Lindau (VHL) syndrome or *SDHB* mutation). MIBG is usually required for most of the extra-adrenal PGL and intra-adrenal PH tumours >5 cm to confirm the tumour.

31. B. Patients with PH may have paroxysmal or persistent hypertension, although blood pressure at the time of diagnosis may be normal in about 10%. The following characteristics should prompt screening for a possible underlying diagnosis of PH or PGL:

- A family history of MEN-2 syndrome, VHL syndrome, or *SDHB* or *SDHB* mutation.
- Detection of an incidental adrenal lesion.
- Orthostatic hypotension (in absence of medication).
- Refractory or paroxysmal hypertension.

Pacak K, Eisenhofer G, Ahlman H, et al. Pheochromocytoma: recommendations for clinical practice from the First International Symposium. Nature Clinical Practice Endocrinology & Metabolism, 2007; 3: 92–102.

32. A. A false positive 24-hour urinary catecholamine measurement as measured with HPLC may be due to factors shown in Table 4.6.

Table 4.6 Factors associated with false positive 24-hour catecholamine results

Medications	Dietary factors	Pathologies
Acetaminophen	Caffeinated drinks	Acute cerebrovascular accident
Amphetamine	Nicotine	Acute heart failure
Cocaine	Bananas	Eclampsia
β-blockers	Pepper	Myocardial infarction
Ephedrine, pseudoephederine		Neuroendocrine tumours
Tricyclic antidepressants		
Levadopa, methyldopa		

Acetaminophen, codeine, metoclopramide, levadopa, labetolol, and peppers may lead to confounding peaks on HPLC chromatography.

Tierney L, Saint S, McPhee S, et al. Current medical diagnosis and treatment. McGraw Hill, 2003.

33. C. MEN-2 is associated with the development of MTC, PH, and mucosal neuromas, intestinal PGLs, and marfanoid body habitus. Patients should undergo *RET* proto-oncogene mutation analysis.

34. E. VHL is characterized by increased risk of development of retinal, cerebellar, and spinal haemangioblastoma, together with renal cell carcinoma. PH are present in about 15–20% of these patients and mostly noradrenaline-secreting extra-adrenal PGLs. Familial PHs can be caused by one of the germ line mutations shown in Table 4.7.

Table 4.7 Gene abnormalities associated with various intra and extra-adrenal PGLs

Clinical condition	Gene abnormality
MEN- 2	*RET* proto-oncogene mutation
VHL disease	*vHL* tumour suppressor gene mutation
Familial PGL	*SHDB, SDHD, SDHC* gene mutation
Neurofibromatosis Type 1	*NF-1* gene mutation

Chen H, Sippel R, O'Dorisio M, et al. The North American Neuroendocrine Tumor Society Consensus Guideline for the Diagnosis and Management of Neuroendocrine Tumors. Pancreas, 2010; 39: 775–783.

35. E. According to the guidelines issued from the 1st International Symposium on PHs (October, 2005), genetic screening should be individualized and is usually indicated in patients with PH who are/have:

- Aged <50 years.
- Bilateral tumours.
- Malignant tumours.
- Multiple tumours.

Pacak K, Eisenhofer G, Ahlman H, et al. Pheochromocytoma: recommendations for clinical practice from the First International Symposium. Nature Clinical Practice Endocrinology & Metabolism, 2007; 3: 92–102.

36. B. About 20–25% of the PH and PGL are believed to have a familial/genetic origin. Genetic testing is not indicated for every gene in every patient with PH. The tumour location, presence of metastasis, and type of catecholamine produced by the tumour cells should be taken into consideration, while requesting genetic analysis for a patient with PH or PGL.

Characteristic features of intra- and extra-adrenal PGLs are as shown in Table 4.8.

Table 4.8 Characteristic features of various familial intra- and extra-adrenal PGLs

Clinical characteristics	MEN-2	SDHB	SDHD	VHL
Location	Adrenal	Extra-adrenal	Head and neck	Adrenal, as well as extra-adrenal
Hormone	Mostly adrenaline	Noradrenaline, dopamine	Usually none or dopamine	Mostly noradrenaline
Metastasis	Rare	>60%	Rare	2–3%

Chen H, Sippel R, O'Dorisio M, et al. The North American Neuroendocrine Tumor Society Consensus Guideline for the Diagnosis and Management of Neuroendocrine Tumors. Pancreas, 2010; 39: 775–783.

Pacak K, Eisenhofer G, Ahlman H, et al. Pheochromocytoma: recommendations for clinical practice from the First International Symposium. Nature Clinical Practice Endocrinology & Metabolism, 2007; 3: 92–102.

37. D. Succinate dehydrogenase subunit D (*SDHD*) gene mutation is mostly associated with head and neck parasympathetic PGLs, while patients with succinate dehydrogenase B subunit (*SDHB*) gene mutation are more likely to present with extra-adrenal disease, bilateral tumours, and metastatic disease.

38. A. Patients with clinically-suspected PH and PGL should undergo plasma or urinary metanephrine measurement as an initial screening procedure. Localization studies should only be arranged if there is reasonable clinical and/or biochemical evidence of a tumour. CT and MRI are usually the initial radiological modalities used to localize the tumour, although these are not specific to identify a mass as a PH or PGL. Functional imaging using ^{131}I-labelled meta-iodobenzylguanide (MIBG) is the modality of choice to confirm the presence of a PH or PGL, and/or assess for metastasis.

Chen H, Sippel R, O'Dorisio M, et al. The North American Neuroendocrine Tumor Society Consensus Guideline for the Diagnosis and Management of Neuroendocrine Tumors. Pancreas, 2010; 39: 775–783.

Pacak K, Eisenhofer G, Ahlman H, et al. Pheochromocytoma: recommendations for clinical practice from the First International Symposium. Nature Clinical Practice Endocrinology & Metabolism, 2007; 3: 92–102.

39. A. Excess catecholamines secreted by PH can precipitate hypertensive crisis by their action on α-adrenergic receptors that induce vasoconstriction. Therefore, adequate α-adrenergic receptor blockage is essential to prevent intra-operative hypertensive crisis due to sudden release of catecholamines into the circulation during handling of the tumour.

The presence of nasal stuffiness and orthostatic hypotension in this patient is consistent with an adequate α-blockage. A β-blocker such as propanolol (non-cardioselective) or metoprolol (cardioselective) can be added if patients develop tachycardia after α-blockage. β-blocker therapy should only be started once adequate α-adrenergic blockage has been achieved.

Pacak K, Linehan W, Eisenhofer G, et al. Recent advances in genetics, diagnosis, localization and treatment of phaeochromocytoma. Annals of Internal Medicine, 2001; 134: 315–329.

Young W. Adrenal causes of hypertension: phaeochromocytoma and primary hyperaldosteronism. Review of Endocrine & Metabolic Disorders, 2007; 8: 309–320.

40. A. ^{131}I-labelled MIBG is usually not required for intra-adrenal tumours (PH) measuring <5 cm (with significant increase in metadrenaline levels), as smaller tumours are rarely associated with metastasis and adrenaline-producing tumours are almost always of adrenal origin.

Genetic screening for *SDHD, SDHB, RET* proto-oncogene, and *VHL* mutation is not indicated in every patient presenting with features of PH or PGL. The tumour location, presence of metastasis and type of catecholamine produced by the tumour cells should be taken into consideration when requesting genetic analysis for a patient with PH

41. E. Autoimmune adrenalitis remains the commonest cause of primary adrenal insufficiency in the developed world. It is characterized by small and atrophic adrenal glands with a thickened capsule, although the medulla is usually preserved. It may be associated with other autoimmune conditions, such as primary autoimmune thyroid disease, coeliac disease, vitiligo, and alopecia areata. These patients may have antibodies to 21-hydroxylase enzyme.

Chakera A and Vaidya B. Addison disease in adults: diagnosis and management. American Journal of Medicine, 2010; 123(5): 409–413.

Ten S, New M, and Maclaren N. Clinical review 130: Addison's disease. Journal of Clinical Endocrinology & Metabolism, 2001; 86(7): 2909–2222.

42. B. In the circulation, about 75% of cortisol is bound to cortisol-binding globulin (CBG) and 15% to albumin. The free cortisol is the biologically active form under regulation of ACTH. The CtBG and albumin levels are reduced in conditions such as cirrhosis and nephrotic syndrome, leading to reduced total cortisol levels as measured by the short synacthen test. Salivary cortisol measurement after stimulation with ACTH may provide a relatively more accurate assessment of hypothalamic–pituitary–adrenal axis in such clinical scenarios as it measures free cortisol.

Thevenot T, Borot S, Remy-Martin A, et al. Assessment of adrenal function in cirrhotic patients using concentration of serum-free and salivary cortisol. Liver International 2011; 31(3): 425–433.

43. E. Adrenoleukodystrophy is an X-linked disorder (due to mutation of the *ABCD1* gene) characterized by high levels of VLCFAs, which accumulate in the brain, adrenal cortex, and liver. It may manifest as neurological symptoms (e.g. cognitive impairment, behavioural problems, gait, and visual disturbance) and primary adrenal insufficiency at a young age. The presence of neurological symptoms in a young man with adrenal insufficiency warrants measurement of VLCFAs to establish the diagnosis.

Moser H, Mahmood A, and Raymond G. X-linked adrenoleukodystrophy. Nature Clinical Practice Neurology 2007; 3: 140–151.

Moser HW. Adrenoleukodystrophy: phenotype, genetics, pathogenesis and therapy. Brain, 1997: 120: 1485–1508.

44. A. Cushing's syndrome can present with a wide spectrum of clinical manifestations, which may be seen in conditions leading to hypercortosolism, such as depression, alcoholism, obesity, and poorly-controlled diabetes. The following clinical features are considered to be more discriminatory for Cushing's syndrome (although not highly sensitive):

• Easy bruisability.
• Facial plethora.
• Proximal myopathy.
• Reddish-purple striae.
• Retardation of growth velocity and weight gain in children.

Nieman L, Biller B, Findling J, et al. The diagnosis of Cushing's syndrome: an Endocrine Society Clinical Practice Guidelines. Journal of Clinical Endocrinology & Metabolism, 2008; 93(5): 1526–1540.

45. A. The dexamethasone suppression test should not be used in patients with epilepsy who are taking medications that increase dexamethasone clearance (see Table 4.9). Measurement of urinary or salivary cortisol in this scenario provides relatively more accurate results.

Table 4.9 Medications that may interfere with diagnostic tests for Cushing's syndrome.

Inducers of hepatic enzymes (increased dexamethasone clearance)	Impaired dexamethasone clearance	Increase in CBG (false positive cortisol results)	Increase urinary free cortisol (UFC)
Carbamazepine	Diltiazem	Oral contraceptive pills	Carbenoxolone
Phenytoin	Fluoxetine	Mitotane	Fenofibrate
Phenobarbiturates	Itraconazole		Liquorice
Primidone	Ritonavir		
Rifampicin			

Gilbert R and Lim E. The diagnosis of Cushing's syndrome: An Endocrine Society Clinical Practice Guideline. Clinical Biochemist Reviews, 2008; 29(3): 103–106.

46. A. The concentration of cortisol binding globulins is increased by oestrogen use, therefore false positive dexamethasone test results are seen in about 50% of women taking the oral contraceptive pills. The urinary or salivary free cortisol measurement is a relatively more accurate screening test for Cushing's syndrome in patients on oestrogen-based medications.

Nieman L, Biller B, Findling J, et al. The diagnosis of Cushing's syndrome: an Endocrine Society Clinical Practice Guidelines. Journal of Clinical Endocrinology & Metabolism, 2008; 93(5): 1526–1540.

47. B. The salivary glands express 11β-hydroxysteroid dehydrogenase type 2 (11β-SD2) enzyme, which plays a role in conversion of biologically-active cortisol to inactive cortisone. Patients using liquorice and/or chewing tobacco may have false positive salivary cortisol results due to inhibition of 11β-SD2.

Salivary cortisol concentration is unaffected by the rate of saliva production and the test results are relatively unaffected by CBG levels (as free cortisol levels are measured).

Gilbert R and Lim E. The diagnosis of Cushing's syndrome: an Endocrine Society Clinical Practice Guideline. Clinical Biochemist Reviews, 2008; 29(3): 103–106.

48. A. The dexamethasone suppression test in pregnancy is associated with high rates of false positive results. The urinary free cortisol excretion remains normal in first trimester of pregnancy and increased up to 3-fold in the second and third trimesters. As a result, a UFC value of more than three times the normal limit is considered suggestive of a diagnosis of Cushing's syndrome in pregnancy. The diagnostic threshold of salivary cortisol values in pregnancy are yet to be validated.

Guignat L and Bertherat J. The diagnosis of Cushing's syndrome: an Endocrine Society Clinical Practice Guidelines: commentary from European perspective. European Journal of Endocrinology, 2010; 163(1): 9–13.

Nieman L, Biller B, Findling J, et al. The diagnosis of Cushing's syndrome: an Endocrine Society Clinical Practice Guidelines. Journal of Clinical Endocrinology & Metabolism, 2008; 93(5): 1526–1540.

49. E. This young man has features of Cushing's syndrome—multiple skin lentigines and atrial myxomas suggestive of an underlying diagnosis of Carney complex, which is usually characterized by:

- Primary pigmented nodular adrenocortical disease (PPNAD).
- Lentigines and spotty pigmentation of face/trunk.
- Myxomas of the heart, skin, and breast.
- GH producing adenoma.
- Sertoli cell tumour.
- Thyroid nodules.

Reynen K. Cardiac myxomas. New England Journal of Medicine, 1995; 333(24): 1610–1617.

Vezzosi D, Vignaux O, Dupin N, and Bertherat J. Carney complex: clinical and genetic 2010 update. Annals of Endocrinology (Paris), 2010; 71(6): 486–493.

50. C. Non-classic congenital adrenal hyperplasia (NCCAH) is characterized by partial deficiency of 21-hydroxylase, leading to features similar to polycystic ovarian syndrome (menstrual irregularities, hirsutism). The diagnosis is based on measurement of 17-OHP. If there is a borderline elevation of 17-OHP levels (5–15 nmol/L) a short synacthen test should be arranged with measurement of 17-OHP levels to confirm or refute the diagnosis.

Speiser P, Azziz R, Baskin L, et al. Congenital adrenal hyperplasia due to steroid 21-hydroxylase deficiency: an Endocrine Society Clinical Practice Guideline. Journal of Clinical Endocrinology & Metabolism, 2010; 95(9): 4133–4160.

51. A. The elevated 17-hydroxyprogesterone (17-OHP) and PRA results in this young man with classic-CAH, despite being on physiological replacement dose of prednisolone and fludrocortisone is indicative of issues with compliance with the medications. Men with classic-CAH are prone to develop testicular adrenal rest tumours, which may not be detected with manual palpation. An ultrasound of testis should be arranged in patients with classic-CAH especially if there is history of poor compliance with the medication.

Speiser P, Azziz R, Baskin L, et al. Congenital adrenal hyperplasia due to steroid 21-hydroxylase deficiency: an Endocrine Society Clinical Practice Guideline. Journal of Clinical Endocrinology & Metabolism, 2010; 95(9); 4133–4160.

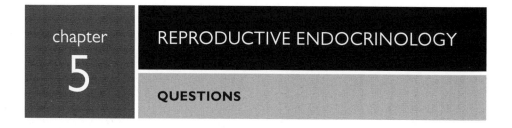
1. **Testis, adrenal glands, and peripheral tissues are the main contributors of circulating sex steroids, including testosterone, dihydrotestosterone, oestradiol, and dehydroepiandrosterone (DHEA) in men.**

   Which one of the following sex steroids is mainly produced by adrenal glands?

   A. Dehydroepiandrosterone
   B. Dihydrotestosterone
   C. Oestradiol
   D. Oestrone
   E. Testosterone

2. **Oestrone and oestradiol in men are primarily derived from peripheral conversion of androstenedione and testosterone, respectively.**

   Which one of the following enzymes is involved in the peripheral conversion of androgens to oestrogens?

   A. 5α-reductase
   B. 21α-hydroxylase
   C. 17-hydroxylase
   D. Aromatase
   E. DHEA sulphate

3. **Testosterone circulates mostly bound to sex hormone-binding globulin (SHBG) or albumin, with only <2% of the free testosterone being biologically active. The SHBG concentrations can be influenced by a variety of medications and clinical conditions, thereby having an impact on serum total testosterone measurement.**

   Which one of the following is associated with an increase in SHBG levels?

   A. Acromegaly
   B. Cushing's syndrome
   C. Exogenous anabolic steroids
   D. Hyperthyroidism
   E. Obesity

4. **Which one of the following is the correct statement regarding the physiological development of gonads?**
    A. The default position of the foetus is to develop into the male sex
    B. The foetal gonads start to differentiate by the fourth week of gestation
    C. The Müllerian ducts develop into the lower part of vagina
    D. The *SRY* gene on the Y chromosome is the trigger that differentiates primordial cells of the gonadal ridge into the testis
    E. The Wolffian duct develops into the epididymis and seminal vesicles under the influence of anti-Müllerian hormones

5. **A 16-year-old girl was reviewed in the endocrine clinic with clinical features of primary amenorrhoea. She had normal growth with no delay in attaining developmental milestones. She had undergone an inguinal hernia repair as a child and had not suffered from any medical or eating disorders. On examination, she was systemically, well with normal breast development, with sparse axillary and pubic hairs.**

    ```
    Investigations:
      FSH                  5.3 U/L (1.4-18.1)
      LH                   4.0 U/L (3.0-8.0)
      prolactin            425 mU/L (45-375)
      serum testosterone   16 nmol/L (0.6-1.9)
      IGF-1                30 nmol/L (16-118)
    ```

    Which one of the following is the probable diagnosis based on her clinical profile?
    A. Adrenal or ovarian carcinoma
    B. Androgen insensitivity syndrome
    C. Exogenous anabolic steroid abuse
    D. Non-classic congenital adrenal hyperplasia
    E. Pituitary germinoma

6. **A 16-year-old girl was reviewed in the endocrine clinic with clinical features of primary amenorrhoea. She had normal growth with no delay in attaining developmental milestones. She had undergone an inguinal hernia repair as a child and had not suffered from any medical or eating disorders. On examination, she was systemically well with normal breast development, with sparse axillary and pubic hairs.**

```
Investigations:
   FSH                  5.3 U/L (1.4-18.1)
   LH                   4.0 U/L (3.0-8.0)
   prolactin            425 mU/L (45-375)
   serum testosterone   16 nmol/L (0.6-1.9)
   IGF-1                30 nmol/L (16-118)
```

All of the following are correct statements regarding her underlying condition except?

A. Gonadectomy should be offered before puberty

B. Hormone replacement therapy has a limited role in management

C. Karyotype may be helpful in establishing the diagnosis

D. Müllerian duct remnants may be recognized on ultrasound.

E. A small uterus may be seen on ultrasound

7. **A 15-year-old girl was referred to the endocrine clinic by her primary care physician with features of primary amenorrhea. She had normal growth and no delay in attaining developmental milestones. Apart from a bicuspid aortic valve for which she was under cardiology follow-up, she had no history of any significant medical disorder. On examination, she was 151 cm tall, with a lack of development of secondary sexual characteristics.**

```
Investigations:
   oestradiol    32 pmol/L (77-1145)
   FSH           46 U/L (1.4-18.1)
   LH            44.5 U/L (3.0-8.0)
   prolactin     350 mU/L (45-375)
   testosterone  1.2 nmol/L (0.6-1.9)
   free T4       8.5 pmol/L (11.5-22.7)
   TSH           7.4 mU/L (0.35-5.5)
```

Which one of the following is the most likely diagnosis, based on her clinical profile?

A. Autoimmune hypothyroidism

B. Kallmann syndrome

C. Klinefelter's syndrome

D. Noonan syndrome

E. Turner's syndrome

8. **A 16-year-old girl was referred to the endocrine clinic by her primary care physician with features of primary amenorrhea. She had normal growth and no delay in attaining developmental milestones. Apart from a bicuspid aortic valve, for which she was under cardiology follow-up, she had no history of any significant medical disorder. On examination, she was 151 cm tall, with a lack of development of secondary sexual characteristics.**

    ```
    Investigations:
        oestradiol      32 pmol/L (77-1145)
        FSH             46 U/L (1.4-18.1)
        LH              44.5 U/L (3.0-8.0)
        prolactin       350 mU/L (45-375)
        testosterone    1.2 nmol/L (0.6-1.9)
        free T4         8.5 pmol/L (11.5-22.7)
        TSH             7.4 mU/L (0.35-5.5)
    ```

    Which one of the following statements regarding her underlying condition is correct?

    A. Arrange endoscopy at diagnosis
    B. Arrange ultrasound of renal tract at diagnosis
    C. Formal audiology assessment at age 1 year and on a 10-yearly interval
    D. GH should be used after puberty
    E. Start oestrogen replacement therapy once diagnosis is established

9. **A 15-year-old boy was referred to the endocrine clinic due to his short stature (155 cm) and delayed puberty. He had a sister who had attained puberty at 12 years of age. His father and mother had a height of 172 and 165 cm, respectively. He had not suffered from any systemic illness or anosmia. On examination, he had sparse body and pubic hair, and his phallus size was small, with testes measuring 4 mL in size bilaterally.**

    ```
    Investigations:
        FSH             3.3 U/L (1.4-18.1)
        LH              4.0 U/L (3.0-8.0)
        testosterone    5.8 nmol/L (8-32)
        prolactin       425 mU/L (45-375)
    ```

    Which one of the following is the probable diagnosis, based on his clinical profile?

    A. Congenital GnRH deficiency
    B. Constitutional delay in puberty
    C. Kallmann syndrome
    D. Klinefelter's syndrome
    E. Noonan syndrome

10. **A 15-year-old boy was referred to endocrine clinic due to his short stature (155cms) and delayed puberty. He had a sister who had attained puberty at 12 years of age. His father and mother had a height of 172 and 165 cm, respectively. He had not suffered from any systemic illness or anosmia. On examination, he had sparse body and pubic hair. The phallus size was small, with testes measuring 4 mL in size bilaterally.**

```
Investigations:
  FSH            3.3 U/L (1.4-18.1)
  LH             4.0 U/L (3.0-8.0)
  Testosterone   5.8 nmol/L (8-32)
  Prolactin      425 mU/L (45-375)
```

Which one of the following is the most appropriate next step in his management?

A. hCG injections

B. Observation

C. Pulsatile GnRH therapy

D. Testosterone 100 mg IM every 2 weeks

E. Testosterone 250 mg IM every 4 weeks

11. **An 18-year-old boy was referred to the endocrine clinic due to lack of libido and delayed puberty. His two elder brothers had attained puberty at 13 and 14 years, respectively. On examination, he was 170 cm tall, with a lack of pubic, axillary, and body hair. His phallus size was 4 cm with a testis volume of 4.5 mL bilaterally. He had features of anosmia and synkinesis.**

```
Investigations:
  FSH            <0.5 U/L (1.4-18.1)
  LH             <0.5 U/L (3.0-8.0)
  prolactin      158 mU/L (45-375)
  testosterone   2.3 nmol/L (8-32)
  free T4        17.1 pmol/L (11.5-22.7)
  TSH            3.8 mU/L (0.35-5.5)
```

Which one of the following proteins is defective in this condition?

A. Ankyrin

B. Anosmin

C. Fibronectin

D. Hyposmin

E. Spectrin

12. **An 18-year-old boy was referred to the endocrine clinic due to lack of libido and delayed puberty. His two elder brothers had attained puberty at 13 and 14 years, respectively. On examination, he was 170 cm tall with a lack of pubic, axillary, and body hair. His phallus size was 4 cm, with a testis volume of 4.5 mL bilaterally. He had features of anosmia and synkinesis.**

```
Investigations:
    FSH            <0.5 U/L  (1.4-18.1)
    LH             <0.5 U/L  (3.0-8.0)
    prolactin      158 mU/L  (45-375)
    testosterone   2.3 nmol/L  (8-32)
    free T4        17.1 pmol/L  (11.5-22.7)
    TSH            3.8 mU/L  (0.35-5.5)
```

All of the following gene mutations cause anosmia or hyposmia in association with hypogonadotrophic hypogonadism except?

A. *FGFR1*

B. *GPR54*

C. *KAL1*

D. *NELF*

E. *PROK2*

13. **A 19-year-old boy was referred to the endocrine clinic due to delayed puberty and a lack of secondary sexual characteristic development. He had no history of systemic illness or delayed attainment of developmental milestones. He had a previous history of surgery for a cleft palate. There was no family history of a constitutional delay in growth. On examination, he was 168 cm tall, with an absence of facial or body hair. His phallus size was 2 cm, with a testis volume of 4.0 mL.**

```
Investigations:
    FSH            <0.5 U/L  (1.4-18.1)
    LH             <0.5 U/L  (3.0-8.0)
    prolactin      302 mU/L  (45-375)
    testosterone   1.5 nmol/L  (8-32)
```

A diagnosis of hypogonadotrophic hypogonadism due to idiopathic or genetic mutation is considered, and genetic analysis is arranged.

Which one of the following is the most appropriate management approach if he desires a family in near future?

A. Anabolic steroids

B. hCG

C. Intra-cytoplasmic sperm injection

D. Intra-uterine insemination

E. Testosterone replacement

14. **A 19-year-old boy was referred to the endocrine clinic due to delayed puberty and a lack of secondary sexual characteristic development. He had no history of systemic illness or delayed attainment of developmental milestones. He had a previous history of surgery for a cleft palate. There was no family history of constitutional delay in growth. On examination, he was 168 cm tall with an absence of facial or body hair. His phallus size was 2cm, with a testis volume of 4.0 mL.**

```
Investigations:
   FSH              <0.5 U/L (1.4-18.1)
   LH               <0.5 U/L (3.0-8.0)
   prolactin        302 mU/L (45-375)
   testosterone     1.5 nmol/L (8-32)
```

A diagnosis of hypogonadotrophic hypogonadism due to KAL1 mutation is confirmed and he was started on hCG therapy.

Which one of the following is a predictor of treatment success with hCG therapy?

A. Absence of sexual maturation

B. Higher baseline testicular volume

C. Higher pre-therapy LH and FSH levels

D. History of cryptorchidism

E. Previous testosterone replacement therapy

15. **A 42-year-old man presented to the endocrine clinic with a gradual decrease in libido and erectile dysfunction. He had back-ground history of type 2 diabetes and dyslipidaemia, and was on metformin, GLP-1 analogues, and atorvastatin therapy. On examination, he had a BMI of 35 kg/m², with central obesity.**

```
Investigations:
   FSH              1.5 U/L (1.4-18.1)
   LH               3.2 U/L (3.0-8.0)
   testosterone     5.8 nmol/L (8-32)
```

All of the following are associated with hypogonadotrophic hypogonadism except?

A. Cushing's disease

B. Haemochromatosis

C. Hyperprolactinaemia

D. Kallmann syndrome

E. Klinefelter's syndrome

16. **A 24-year-old professional rugby player was referred to the endocrine clinic with features of a lack of libido and erectile dysfunction. He had no history of systemic illness or weight loss. He denied the use of anabolic steroids or recreational drugs. On examination, he had a muscular build and a BMI of 28 kg/m². He had normal secondary sexual characteristics with no anosmia.**

```
Investigations:
   FSH           1.2 U/L  (1.4-18.1)
   LH            2.5 U/L  (3.0-8.0)
   testosterone  4.0 nmol/L (8-32)
```

Which one of the following clinical features is indicative of the origin of hypogonadism in the pre-pubertal age group?

A. Infertility

B. Gynaecomastia

C. Low libido

D. Testes volume <6 cm³

E. Thinning of facial and axillary hair

17. **High-amplitude pulses of GnRH are believed to play a key role in onset of puberty in both sexes.**

All of the following stages of puberty are under the influence of GnRH except?

A. Growth spurt

B. Menarche

C. Pubarche

D. Thelarche

E. None of the above

18. **A 24-year-old woman presented to the endocrine clinic with secondary amenorrhoea for the previous 18 months. She had experienced night sweats, hot flushes and pain while having sexual intercourse over the previous 6 months. She had a background history of pernicious anaemia and type 1 diabetes. On examination, she had a height of 171 cm with a BMI of 22 kg/m². She had no features of proximal myopathy or stria.**

```
Investigations:
    oestradiol    32 pmol/L (77-1145)
    FSH           29 U/L (1.4-18.1)
    LH            25.1 U/L (3.0-8.0)
    prolactin     302 mU/L (45-375)
    testosterone  1.1 nmol/L (0.6-1.9)
```

Which one of the following is the probable diagnosis, based on her clinical profile?

A. Kallmann syndrome

B. Noonan syndrome

C. Polycystic ovarian disease

D. Premature ovarian failure

E. Turner's syndrome

19. **A 22-year-old woman was referred to the endocrine clinic, with a 3-month history of amenorrhoea and elevated prolactin levels. She also complained of headache, fatigue, and non-specific abdominal pain. She had a background medical history of depression and had been on citalopram tablets. On examination, she had a BMI of 26 kg/m², with facial puffiness and central obesity. Her visual fields were normal on confrontation.**

```
Investigations:
    oestradiol    1488 pmol/L (77-1145)
    FSH           2.5 U/L (1.4-18.1)
    LH            3.2 U/L (3.0-8.0)
    prolactin     1505 mU/L (45-375)
    testosterone  3.1 nmol/L (0.6-1.9)
```

Which one of the following is the most appropriate next investigation in her clinical scenario?

A. Domeperidone test

B. MRI pituitary

C. Short synacthen test

D. Urinary free cortisol measurement

E. Urine for pregnancy test

20. **A 28-year-old female company executive was referred to the endocrine clinic by her GP, with secondary amenorrhoea for the previous 18 months. She had a busy lifestyle, and did regular aerobic exercise and long distance running. On examination, she had a BMI of 18 kg/m^2, with normal secondary sexual characteristics and no features of hirsutism.**

```
Investigations:
   oestradiol              24 pmol/L (77-1145)
   FSH                     1.8 U/L (1.4-18.1)
   LH                      4.5 U/L (3.0-8.0)
   prolactin               220 mU/L (45-375)
   testosterone            1.6 nmol/L (0.6-1.9)
   urine for pregnancy test  negative
```

Which one of the following is a feature associated with her underlying condition?

A. Dyspareunia

B. Higher risk of breast carcinoma

C. Higher risk of endometrial carcinoma

D. High leptin levels

E. Regular ovulation

21. **A 17-year-old girl was referred to endocrine clinic with features of menstrual irregularity, and increased facial and body hair. She had attained menarche at the age of 13 years and had normal secondary sexual characteristic development. She was in a stable relationship and was using a barrier method of contraception. On examination, she had a BMI of 32 kg/m^2, with increased facial and body hair. There were no clinical features of proximal myopathy or easy bruisability.**

```
Investigations:
   oestradiol     115 pmol/L (77-1145)
   FSH            3.2 U/L (1.4-18.1)
   LH             9.1 U/L (3.0-8.0)
   prolactin      355 mU/L (45-375)
   testosterone   2.2 nmol/L (0.6-1.9)
```

Which one of the following is the most appropriate management option for her menstrual irregularity?

A. Cyproterone acetate

B. Eflornithine

C. Metformin

D. Oral contraceptive pills

E. Spiranolactone

22. **A 25-year-old woman was on Depo Provera® (depot medroxy progesterone, DMPA) for contraception over the previous 2 years. She was a non-smoker with no significant past medical history.**

    All of the following are true statements regarding the use of DMPA except?

    A. Associated intermittent bleeds and weight gain.
    B. Associated mild increase in thrombosis risk
    C. Associated reversible bone density
    D. Ensures good long-term efficacy and compliance
    E. Fertility may be delayed by up to 12 months on cessation of DMPA.

23. **A 45-year-old woman presented to the medical clinic with symptoms of mood swings, menstrual irregularities, and hot flushes for the previous 6 months. Her body weight had been stable and there had been no alteration in bowel habits.**

    Which one of the following hormone profile is consistent with a peri-menopausal state?

    A. High inhibin
    B. High LH
    C. Low FSH
    D. Low oestradiol
    E. Low progesterone

24. **A couple in their early thirties were reviewed in the infertility clinic. They had been married for 5 years and the wife had failed to conceive, despite unprotected intercourse for previous 18 months. On examination, the husband had a BMI of 23 kg/m^2 with normal secondary sexual characteristics and a testes volume >10 cm^3**

    What percentage of infertility is believed to be due to male-partner related factors?

    A. <5%
    B. 10–15%
    C. 20–25%
    D. 40–45%
    E. >50%

25. **A 25-year-old man was referred to the endocrine clinic with symptoms of erectile dysfunction. He had been in a stable relationship for the previous 18 months and had noticed a low sexual drive. On examination, he was 187cm tall with a BMI of 21 kg/m². He had sparse facial and body hair, with gynaecomastia. His testes were small in volume and firm in consistency on palpation.**

```
Investigations:
    FSH            30.5 U/L  (1.4-18.1)
    LH             35.1 U/L  (3.0-8.0)
    Prolactin      210 mU/L  (45-375)
    Testosterone   1.7 nmol/L (8-32)
```

Which one of the following is usually is the most appropriate management approach in his case?

A. β-hCG therapy
B. GnRH analogues
C. Octeroetide
D. Sildenafil (prn use)
E. Testosterone replacement

26. **A 25-year-old man was referred to the endocrine clinic with symptoms of erectile dysfunction. He had been in a stable relationship for the previous 18 months and had noticed a low sexual drive. On examination, he was 187cm tall with a BMI of 21 kg/m². He had sparse facial and body hair, with gynaecomastia. His testes were small in volume and firm in consistency on palpation.**

```
Investigations:
    FSH            30.5 U/L  (1.4-18.1)
    LH             35.1 U/L  (3.0-8.0)
    Prolactin      210 mU/L  (45-375)
    Testosterone   1.7 nmol/L (8-32)
```

All of the following clinical pathologies may be associated with his underlying condition except?

A. Bronchitis and emphysema
B. Increased incidence of pulmonary embolism
C. Kypho-scoliosis
D. Mitral valve prolapse
E. Osteoporosis

27. **A 25-year-old man was referred to the endocrine clinic for further evaluation of his symptoms of low libido and fatigue. He had no history of any previous medical disorder, except for a bout of severe mumps at 17 years of age. On examination, he was 174 cm tall with a BMI of 22 kg/m². He had bilateral gynaecomastia and scanty body hair, with a testicular volume of 4 mL³.**

    ```
    Investigations:
      FSH            30.9 U/L (1.4-18.1)
      LH             35.7 U/L (3.0-8.0)
      prolactin      154 mU/L (45-375)
      testosterone   1.5 nmol/L (8.4-28.7)
    ```

    He was keen to assess his fertility status and discussed further management approach.

    Which one of the following is the most suitable approach for the management of his infertility?

    A. β-hCG

    B. GnRH

    C. In vitro fertilization

    D. Octreotide

    E. Testosterone replacement

28. **A 26-year-old woman was referred to the endocrine clinic for further evaluation of her symptoms of menstrual irregularity, acne, and excessive facial hair growth. On examination, she had a BMI of 30 kg/m² with no features of Cushing's syndrome.**

    Her biochemical investigations and ultrasound pelvis results were consistent with a diagnosis of polycystic ovarian syndrome (PCOS).

    Which one of the following investigations can be used to assess her ovulatory function?

    A. Follicular 17-hydroxy progesterone

    B. Follicular 21-hydroxy progesterone

    C. Mid-luteal 17-hydroxy progesterone

    D. Mid-luteal 21-hydroxy progesterone

    E. Mid-luteal oestradiol

29. **A 35-year-old woman was referred to the endocrine clinic with a 6-week history of rapidly progressive facial and body hair. She had also developed secondary amenorrhoea for last 3 months. On examination, she had a BMI of 25 kg/m², with features of excessive hair growth involving the face, upper back, lower abdomen, and legs (Ferriman–Gallway score of 16).**

    Investigations:
       FSH   3.5 U/L (follicular 0.5-5, mid-cycle 8-33,
                      luteal 2-8)
       LH   8.8 U/L (follicular 3-12, mid-cycle 20-80,
                      luteal 3-16)
       oestradiol   120 pmol/L (follicular 17-260, luteal 180-1100)
       prolactin   145 mU/L (60-560)
       testosterone   12.5 nmol/L (0.6-1.9)

    Which one of the following is the most appropriate investigation, based on her clinical profile?

    A. CT of the abdomen and pelvis
    B. Genetic counselling
    C. Karyotype analysis
    D. MRI pituitary
    E. Octreotide scan

30. **A 26-year-old woman was referred to the endocrine clinic for evaluation and management of her long-standing excessive facial hair growth. She had no history of galactorrhoea, menstrual disturbance headaches, or weight gain. She was on long-term anti-epileptics for idiopathic epilepsy. On examination, she had a BMI of 28 kg/m² with no features of proximal myopathy or easy bruisability.**

    Investigations:
       FSH   4.5 U/L (follicular 0.5-5, mid-cycle 8-33,
                      luteal 2-8)
       LH   4.8 U/L (follicular 3-12, mid-cycle 20-80,
                      luteal 3-16)
       oestradiol   163 pmol/L (follicular 17-260, luteal 180-1100)
       prolactin   280 mU/L (60-560)
       testosterone   1.4 nmol/L (0.6-1.9)

    Which one of the following is the most likely aetiology for her hirsutism, based on her clinical profile?

    A. Iatrogenic
    B. Idiopathic
    C. Non-classic congenital adrenal hyperplasia
    D. Polycystic ovarian disease
    E. Pregnancy

31. **A 25-year-old woman was referred to the endocrine clinic with a history of menstrual irregularities and excessive hair growth on face. On examination, she had a BMI of 32 kg/m² with no clinical features of proximal myopathy or easy bruisability.**

    Which one of the following blood results is consistent with a diagnosis of polycystic ovarian disease?

    A. Low 17-hydroxy progesterone levels
    B. Low prolactin levels
    C. Raised FSH levels
    D. Raised SHBG levels
    E. Raised testosterone levels

32. **A 35-year-old woman was reviewed in the endocrine clinic for her symptoms of excessive facial and body hair growth. She had menarche at age 13 years and had suffered from dysmenorrhoea for the last two decades, for which she had been on oral contraceptive pills. She was in a steady relationship and was not keen to start a family.**

    On examination, she had a BMI of 32 kg/m², with excessive facial and body hair. There were no features of proximal myopathy or easy bruisability.

    ```
    Investigations:
       FSH                9.5 U/L (follicular 0.5-5, mid-cycle 8-33,
                          luteal 2-8)
       LH                 15.1 U/L (follicular 3-12, mid-cycle 20-80,
                          luteal 3-16)
       Oestradiol         105 pmol/L (follicular 17-260, luteal 180-1100)
       Prolactin          220 mU/L (60-560)
       Testosterone       2.2 nmol/L (0.6-1.9)
    ```

    An ultrasound pelvis showed the presence of multiple ovarian cysts.

    Which one of the following is the most appropriate therapeutic approach to manage her hirsutism?

    A. Clomiphene
    B. Ethinyl oestradiol
    C. Metformin
    D. Observation
    E. Spironolactone

33. **A 52-year-old man with Klinefelter's syndrome was reviewed in the endocrine clinic for a routine follow-up visit. He complained of symptoms of feeling generally unwell, back pain, and weight loss. He had been on testosterone replacement therapy since his early teenage years.**

Investigations:
```
FSH                  22.5 U/L (1.4-18.1)
LH                   30.1 U/L (3.0-8.0)
prolactin            350 mU/L (45-375)
testosterone         7.4 nmol/L (8.4-28.7)
corrected calcium    2.9 mmol/L (2.4-2.62)
```

Which one of the following is the most appropriate next step in his management?

A. Bone scan

B. Breast examination

C. CT abdomen and pelvis

D. Digital examination of prostate

E. Myeloma screen

34. **A 25-year-old professional body-builder was referred to the endocrine clinic with erectile dysfunction. He admitted to having used anabolic steroids and testosterone to help build his muscle mass, although he had stopped using these 6 weeks previously. He had reached puberty at 13 years of age and had normal libido till about 1 year ago. On examination, he had a BMI of 27 kg/m² with a muscular build. He had normal secondary sexual characteristics and no features of anosmia.**

Investigations:
```
FSH              <0.5 U/L (1.4-18.1)
LH               <0.5 U/L (3.0-8.0)
prolactin        550 mU/L (45-375)
testosterone     3.5 nmol/L (8.4-28.7)
```

Which one of the following is the most appropriate management approach in his case?

A. β-hCG therapy

B. MRI pituitary

C. Repeat hormone profile in 12 weeks

D. Phosphodiesterase 5 inhibitors

E. Testosterone therapy

35. **A 21-year-old woman, of Mexican origin, was referred to the endocrinology clinic with a 3-year history of excessive body hair growth and menstrual irregularities. On examination, she had excessive hair covering below the lower lip, chin, lower abdomen, and arms.**

Investigations:
```
FSH                  5.5 U/L (follicular 0.5-5, mid-cycle
                     8-33, luteal 2-8)
LH                   7.8 U/L (follicular 3-12, mid-cycle 20-80,
                     luteal 3-16)
oestradiol           62 pmol/L (follicular 17-260, luteal
                     180-1100)
testosterone         0.3 nmol/L (<0.5)
17-OH progesterone   12.5 nmol/L (1-5)
```

Which one of the following is the most appropriate investigation to confirm the diagnosis?

A. CT adrenals
B. Karyotype analysis
C. MRI pituitary
D. Short synacthen test (measurement of 17-OH progesterone)
E. Ultrasound ovaries

36. **A 21-year-old woman, of Mexican origin, was referred to the endocrinology clinic with a 3-year history of excessive body hair growth and menstrual irregularities. On examination, she had excessive hair covering the lower lip, chin, lower abdomen, and arms.**

Investigations:
```
FSH                  5.5 U/L (follicular 0.5-5, mid-cycle 8-33,
                     luteal 2-8)
LH                   7.8 U/L (follicular 3-12, mid-cycle 20-80,
                     luteal 3-16)
oestradiol           62 pmol/L (follicular 17-260, luteal
                     180-1100)
testosterone         0.3 nmol/L (<0.5)
17-OH progesterone   45 nmol/L (1-5)
```

Which one of the following is the most appropriate therapeutic management approach in her case?

A. Clomiphene
B. Fludrocortisone
C. Metformin
D. Prednisolone
E. Spironolactone

37. **A 26-year-old lady with congenital adrenal hyperplasia (CAH) was reviewed in the endocrinology clinic, on a routine follow-up visit. She was 8 weeks pregnant, and complained of nausea and morning sickness.**

    Which one of the following is the most appropriate immediate management approach?

    A. Chorionic villous sampling
    B. Genetic counselling
    C. Screen partner for CAH
    D. Start dexamethasone
    E. Ultrasound scan at 20 weeks

38. **A 25-year-old Caucasian man was reviewed in the endocrinology clinic for further evaluation of his infertility. He had a background history of bronchiectesis and dextrocardia. On examination, he had a BMI of 22 kg/m², with clubbing of the nails and bilateral coarse crepitations at the lung bases. He had scanty body and facial hair, and gynaecomastia.**

    ```
    Semen analysis results:
      Semen volume   4 mL
      Sperm count    30 million/mL
      Motility       5%
      Morphology     40% normal
    ```

    Which one of the following treatment plans is most likely to be successful in dealing with infertility in his clinical context?

    A. Anabolic steroids
    B. Epididymovasostomy
    C. Gonadotropins
    D. Intracytoplasmic sperm injection
    E. Testosterone replacement

39. **A 52-year-old man presented to his general practitioner with a history of a progressive decline in libido and lack of energy. He had endured a traumatic injury to the testis and pelvic region in a traffic accident about a year previously. On examination, he had a BMI of 22 kg/m² with normal secondary sexual characteristics.**

```
Investigations:
   FSH                  28.5 U/L (1.4-18.1)
   LH                   23.4 U/L (3.0-8.0)
   serum testosterone   4.2 nmol/L (8-32)
```

He was considered for a trial of testosterone replacement therapy.

Which one of the following is an absolute contraindication for the initiation of testosterone therapy?

A. Benign prostate hyperplasia
B. Breast carcinoma
C. Pituitary apoplexy
D. Polycythaemia
E. Sleep apnoea

40. **A 45-year-old man was referred to the endocrine clinic with a progressive decline in his libido, and difficulty in achieving and maintaining an erection for the previous 6 months. He had a background history of diabetes and dyslipidaemia, for which he was on metformin and statin therapy. On examination, he had a BMI of 42 kg/m² with central obesity, although there was no anosmia or proximal myopathy/ easy bruisability.**

```
Investigations:
   FSH                  2.5 U/L (1.4-18.1)
   LH                   3.5 U/L (3.0-8.0)
   prolactin            355 mU/L (45-375)
   serum testosterone   4.6 nmol/L (8-32)
```

Which one of the following is the most appropriate step in management that can potentially help improve his symptoms of erectile dysfunction?

A. β-hCG
B. Cabergoline
C. GLP-1 analogues
D. Testosterone replacement
E. Weight loss

41. **A 32-year-old man was reviewed in the infertility clinic (with his partner) for the inability of the female partner to conceive, despite having unprotected sexual intercourse for the previous 18 months. Neither partners had a history of any systemic illness and were not on any medications. The general physical and systemic examination of both the partners was unremarkable.**

```
Semen analysis results of male partner:
   semen volume   2.5 mL
   sperm count    14.2 million/mL
   motility       62%
   fructose       195 mg/dL
```

Which one of the following is the correct description of his semen analysis results?

A. Asthenospermia

B. Ejaculatory duct obstruction

C. Normal results

D. Oligospermia

E. Teratospermia

42. **A 24-year-old woman presented with menstrual irregularities and facial hair growth.**

On examination, she had features of hirsutism without any Cushinoid phenotypic features.

```
Investigations:
FSH            5.5 U/L (follicular 0.5-5, mid-cycle 8-33,
               luteal 2-8)
LH             19.1 U/L (follicular 3-12, mid-cycle 20-80,
               luteal 3-16)
oestradiol     92 pmol/L (follicular 17-260, luteal 180-1100)
testosterone   1.4 nmol/L (<0.5)
```

Which one of the following statements is supportive of a diagnosis of PCOS, based on ultrasonography imaging?

A. >5 follicles measuring >15 mm in size

B. Endometrial hyperplasia <5 mm

C. Follicular string of pearl appearance

D. Hypo-echoic central stroma

E. Ovarian size <15 cm³

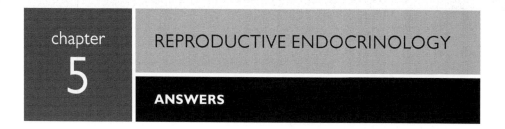

1. A. Testicular secretion contributes to more than 95% of the circulating testosterone levels, while dihydrotestosterone is mostly formed by the peripheral conversion of testosterone by enzyme 5α reductase (see Table 5.1). Oestrone and oestradiol in men are primarily derived from peripheral conversion of androstenedione and testosterone, respectively. DHEA is primarily secreted by the adrenal glands.

Table 5.1 Relative contribution of various organs to sex steroid levels in men

	Testicular secretion	Adrenal secretion	Peripheral conversion
Testosterone	90–95%	<1%	<5%
Dihydrotestosterone	15–20%	<1%	80–85%
Oestradiol	15–20%	<1%	80–85%
Dehydroepiandrosterone	5–10%	90–95%	–

Gardner D and Shoback D. Gardner D and Shoback D. Greenspan's Basic and Clinical Endocrinology (9th edn). McGraw-Hill Medical, 2011.

2. D. Aromatase enzyme is localized in the endoplasmic reticulum and involved in the peripheral conversion of androstenedione and testosterone to oestrone and oestradiol, respectively. It is present in organs such as the brain, adipose tissues, gonads, and skin. An increase in aromatase activity, with the resultant increase in oestrone and oestradiol levels, is believed to be one of the major contributory factors to hypogonadotrophic hypogonadism in obese men.

Grossman M. Low testosterone in men with type 2 diabetes: significance and treatment. Journal of Clinical Endocrinology and Metabolism, 2011; 96(8): 2341–2353.

Guay A. The emerging link between hypogonadism and metabolic syndrome. Journal of Andrology, 2009; 30: 370–376.

3. D. A decrease in SHBG levels may be seen with:

- Acromegaly or GH hormone use.
- Cushing's syndrome.
- Exogenous glucocorticoid or anabolic steroid use.
- Hypothyroidism.
- Obesity.

An increase in SHBG levels may be seen with:

- Cirrhosis.
- Oestrogens.
- Hyperthyroidism.

- Tamoxifen.
- Phenytoin.

Gardner D and Shoback D. Greenspan's Basic and Clinical Endocrinology (9th edn). McGraw-Hill Medical, 2011.

4. D. During the first 7 weeks of foetal development, the gonadal ridge is bi-potential, irrespective of the chromosomal sex. In the presence of the testis determining gene on Y chromosome (*TDY*) or sex differentiation gene on p arm of Y chromosome (*SRY*) primordial cells of gonadal ridge differentiate into testis.

Primordial cells differentiate into the precursors of supporting cells or steroid-secreting gonadal cells. The supporting cell precursors develop into either testis-specific Sertoli cells or ovary-specific follicle (granulosa) cells, depending on the chromosomal sex of the foetus. The precursor of steroid lineage differentiates into steroid-secreting Leydig cells in the testis or Theca cells in the ovary.

Wolffian (mesonephric) ducts are precursors of male reproductive ducts system, while Müllerian (para-mesonephric) ducts are precursors of the female reproductive duct system. Under the influence of anti-Müllerian hormone (AMH) produced by Sertoli cells, the Müllerian ducts regress in males and result in the formation of the epididymis, vas deferens, and seminal vesicles. In the absence of AMH, the Müllerian duct forms the oviduct, uterus, and upper part of vagina.

5. B. Androgen insensitivity syndrome (AIS) is a rare X-linked recessive condition, characterized by partial or complete resistance to androgens. The karyotype of patients with AIS is XY with partial or complete failure of virilization resulting in female external genitalia and undescended testes often presenting as inguinal masses during childhood.

6. D. The presence of secondary sexual characteristics of a female in the presence of elevated male range testosterone levels is suggestive of a diagnosis of androgen insensitivity syndrome (AIS). It is an X-linked disorder characterized by androgen receptor resistance, which leads to complete or partial failure of virilization.

These individuals are usually raised as girls due to their phenotypic appearance and may have female external genitalia. The upper vagina, uterus, and fallopian tubes are characteristically absent. In some patients, the presence of inguinal masses at birth/neonatal period may lead to the subsequent identification of testes during elective surgical procedure.

A few patients may seek medical attention due to the primary amenorrhoea during the adolescent period of life. The testis may be palpable in the inguinal region and should be removed due to the associated high risk of malignancy. Hormone replacement therapy with oestrogens along with psychological support forms the mainstay of medical therapy.

Batch J, Patterson M, Hughes I, et al. Androgen insensitivity syndrome. Reproductive Medicine Review, 1992; 1(2): 131–150.

Gingu C, Dick A, Pătrăşcoiu S, et al. Testicular feminization: complete androgen insensitivity syndrome. Discussions based on a case report. Romanian Journal of Morphology and Embryology. 2014; 55(1): 177–181.

Hughes A, Werner R, Bunch T, et al. Androgen insensitivity syndrome. Seminars in Reproductive Medicine, 2012; 30(05): 432–442.

7. E. Turner's syndrome is characterized by phenotypic features such as short stature, webbed neck (due to extra skin folds), lymphoedema of hands/feet and skeletal abnormalities. The patients may present with primary amenorrhoea or features of primary ovarian failure. The biochemistry is consistent with primary gonadal failure (low oestradiol with elevated LH and FSH levels).

8. B. The clinical features of short stature, congenital heart disease, and primary amenorrhoea due to gonadal failure (elevated gonadotropin s and low oestrogens) are suggestive of a diagnosis of Turner's syndrome (Ullrich–Turner syndrome). Patients should undergo an echocardiography and ultrasound at the time of diagnosis. Formal audiology assessments are recommended at age 1 year and at 5-yearly intervals due to associated sensori-neural hearing loss. GH replacement may be used before puberty and may help to attain gain in linear height. Oestrogen replacement therapy is usually started around age 12–14 years.

Table 5.2 shows the characteristic clinical features associated with this syndrome, and Table 5.3 shows the guidelines regarding the management of Turner's syndrome, based on age.

Table 5.2 Clinical features which may be associated with Turner's syndrome

Genotype	46,X—50%
	46,X/XX mosiacism—20%
	Abnormalities of the X chromosome, such as X fragments, iso-chromosomes or rings—30%
Phenotype	Female
	Web neck, wide-spaced nipples
	Rarely clitoral enlargement if there is translocation of fragments of Y chromosome
Cardiac defects	Bicuspid aortic valve, coarctation of aorta,
Renal defects	Congenital renal malformations
	Recurrent infections
	Nephrocalcinosis
	Hypertension
Growth	Short stature—GH therapy in combination with aromatase inhibitors
Puberty	Delayed/non-progression—low dose oestrogens (1/10th adult dose) at 12 years to initiate puberty and then increase the dose gradually to maintain feminine phenotype.
	Add progestogens to allow for withdrawal bleed.
	Hormone replacement therapy helps to maintain bone health
Fertility	Infertility—ovum donation and in vitro fertilization (IVF) will be helpful in some cases.

Table 5.3 Guidelines regarding management of Turner's syndrome based on age

At diagnosis	Echocardiography
	Ultrasound of abdomen and pelvis
5-yearly	Audiology assessments
Age >7 years	Start GH therapy and monitor response
Age 12–14 years	Oestrogen replacement started
	2 years later start on combined oestrogen and progesterone
	Once puberty is induced, they need follow-up to monitor the hormone replacement therapy (HRT)
	Stop GH if:
	• rate of height gained is <2 cm/year
	• final height attained
	• growth velocity less than 50% gain
	from baseline than predicted

Data from Gwalik A. Treatment of Turner's syndrome during transition. EJE:2014; 170, R57–74.

Carel JC. Growth hormone in Turner syndrome: twenty years after, what can we tell our patients? Journal of Clinical Endocrinology & Metabolism, 2005; 90(6): 3793–3794.

Gwalik A. Treatment of Turner's syndrome during transition. European Journal of Endocrinology, 2014; 170: R57–R74.

9. B. The first sign of puberty in boys is usually an increase in the size and volume of the testes due to a FSH-stimulated increase on seminiferous tubular development. Pubic hair growth takes place as a result of adrenal and testicular androgen secretion. Constitutional delay (CD) is one of the commonest aetiology, leading to short stature and delayed puberty in the adolescent age group. It should be considered if there is a lack of signs of puberty at age 13–15 and 14–16 years in girls and boys, respectively. There is usually a family history of CD. In most of cases, it is not pathological and represents the extreme end of normal physiology. The growth and development of such individuals is appropriate for their skeletal age, rather than chronological age.

Our patient presented with a lack of pubertal development and delayed growth at age 15 years, raising the probability of CD. The differential diagnosis hypogonadotrophic hypogonadism is in view of the low testosterone and inappropriately normal gonadotropin levels.

Harrington J and Palmert M. Distinguishing constitutional delay of growth and puberty from isolated hypogonadotropic hypogonadism: critical appraisal of available diagnostic tests. Journal of Clinical Endocrinology & Metabolism, 2012; 97(9): 3056–3067.

10. B. The most probable diagnosis in this clinical scenario is CD. The immediate step in management includes reassurance to the patient/patient's family and observation. These individuals need to be monitored with frequent (3–6-monthly) growth measurements. Medical treatment is usually not required, although in patients displaying features of psychological stress, exogenous testosterone therapy in low dose (100 mg IM every 4 weeks for 4–6 months) may be used to stimulate the hypothalamic–pituitary–gonadal axis.

Han T and Bouloux P. What is the optimal therapy for young males with hypogonadotropic hypogonadism? Clinical Endocrinology, 2010; 72: 731–737.

11. B. The biochemical profile of hypogonadotrophic hypogonadism (low testosterone and low FSH and LH levels), with the presence of clinical features of anosmia/hyposmia, is suggestive of a diagnosis of Kallmann syndrome in this young individual. It is an X-linked disorder, characterized by mutations in *KAL1* gene, which encodes anosmin, a protein that mediates the migration of neural progenitors of the olfactory bulb and GnRH-producing neurons.

Sato N. Clinical assessment and mutation analysis of Kallmann syndrome 1 (KAL1) and fibroblast growth factor receptor 1 (FGFR1, or KAL2) in five families and 18 sporadic patients. Journal of Clinical Endocrinology & Metabolism, 2004; 89: 1079–1088.

American Association of Clinical Endocrinologists. Medical guidelines for clinical practice for the evaluation and treatment of hypogonadism in adult male patients. 2002 update, AACE Hypogonadism Guidelines. Endocrine Practice, 2002; 8(6): 1–18.

12. B. Hypogonadotrophic hypogonadism and anosmia may be associated with mutations of the *KAL1*, *FGFR1*, *NELF*, and *PROK2* genes. Autosomal recessive mutations in the G protein-coupled receptor gene (*GPR54*) cause gonadotropin deficiency without anosmia (see Table 5.4).

Table 5.4 Genetic mutations associated with hypogonadotrophic hypogonadism

Gene defect	Clinical features
FGFR1	Autosomal dominant
	Ansomia, cleft lip/palate, synkinesis, syndactyly
NELF and PROK2	Autosomal recessive
	Anosmia
GPR54	Autosomal recessive

13. B. hCG or GnRH are considered to be the treatment of choice for hypogonadotrophic hypogonadal men desiring fertility. hCG is given at a dose of 1000–2500 IU twice weekly for a duration of 8–12 weeks. This treatment can lead to an increase in testosterone levels and may induce spermatogenesis in selected patients.

Fraietta R, Zylberstejn D, Esteves S. Hypogonadotropic hypogonadism revisited. Clinics. 2013; 68(S1): 81–88.

Warne D, Decosterd G, Okada H, et al. A combined analysis of data to identify predictive factors for spermatogenesis in men with hypogonadotropic hypogonadism treated with recombinant human follicle-stimulating hormone and human chorionic gonadotropin. Fertility and Sterility, 2009; 92(2): 594–604.

14. B. The following are considered predictors of therapeutic success with hCG therapy:

- A higher baseline testicular volume.
- No history of previous testosterone replacement therapy.

Pre-therapy FSH, LH, and testosterone levels are not considered to be predictors of therapeutic success with hCG therapy.

Farhat R. Outcome of gonadotropin therapy for male infertility due to hypogonadotrophic hypogonadism. Pituitary, 2010; 13(2): 105–110.

Warne D, Decosterd G, Okada H, et al. A combined analysis of data to identify predictive factors for spermatogenesis in men with hypogonadotrophic hypogonadism treated with recombinant human follicle-stimulating hormone and human chorionic gonadotropin. Fertility and Sterility, 2009; 92(2): 594–604.

Zitzmann M. Hormone substitution in male hypogonadism. Molecular and Cellular Endocrinology, 2000; 161(1–2): 73–88.

15. E. The most common aetiologies leading to hypogonadotrophic hypogonadism in clinical practice, include eating disorders such as anorexia nervosa, excessive exercise (e.g. athletes training for long-distance running), increased BMI/morbid obesity, use of anabolic steroids, and genetic disorders such as Kallmann syndrome. See Table 5.5.

Table 5.5 Aetiologies related with hypogonadotrophic hypogonadism

Genetic causes	Endocrine conditions	Miscellaneous causes	Eating disorder
Kallmann syndrome	Hyperprolactinaemia	Haemochromatosis	Increased BMI
Idiopathic	Cushing's disease	Anabolic steroids	Anorexia nervosa
Prader-Willi syndrome	Pituitary lesion/irradiation/surgery	Alcohol/opioids	

Melmed S, Polonsky K, Reed Larsen P, et al. Williams textbook of endocrinology (12th edn). Elsevier, 2011.

16. D. Gynaecomastia, infertility, and low libido may be seen in patients with testosterone deficiency in pre-pubertal, as well as post-pubertal period (see Table 5.6).

Table 5.6 Effect of testosterone deficiency in pre- and post-pubertal age groups

	Pre-pubertal	Post-pubertal
Stature	Eunuchoidal	Normal
Testes	Small (usually <6 cm^3)	Normal /slightly low (>10 cm^3)
Penis	Small (<5 cm)	Normal size
Hair growth	Scanty facial and axillary hair	Thinning of facial and axillary hair
Voice	High pitched	Normal
Prostate	Small	Normal size

17. C. In girls, the various stages of puberty include thelarche (breast development), puberache (pubic hair development), and menarche (onset of menstrual cycles).

Pubarche is not under the influence of GnRH

Melmed S, Polonsky K, Reed Larsen P, et al. Williams textbook of endocrinology (12th edn). Elsevier, 2011.

18. D. Premature ovarian failure is characterized by signs and symptoms of oestrogen deficiency, such as hot flushes, painful intercourse, and dry vagina, with biochemical features of primary hypogonadism (low oestradiol and elevated FSH/LH). It can be autoimmune, iatrogenic (post-irradiation), or idiopathic. The treatment is with oestrogen replacement therapy. Patients are usually infertile and require assisted fertilization. Patients with suspected autoimmune ovarian failure should be screened for adrenal insufficiency and thyroid dysfunction.

Maclaran K and Panay N. Premature ovarian failure. Journal of Family Planning and Reproductive Health Care, 2011; 37: 35–42.

19. E. Pregnancy is associated with the following hormone changes:

- Increase in oestradiol and oestriol levels.
- Reduced LH, FSH levels.
- Increase in testosterone levels while DHEA levels fall.
- Increase in hCG, human placental lactogen (hPL).
- GH and ACTH remain unchanged, TSH levels reach nadir during the first trimester.
- Progesterone levels increase and 17-hydroxy-progesterone peak around week 5.
- Cortisol levels increase.
- Total T4 and T3 levels increase during the first trimester, FT3 and FT4 remain unchanged.

20. A. The combination of low BMI and secondary amenorrhea of >6 months duration is suggestive of a diagnosis of hypothalamic amenorrhoea. It is often seen in association with a stressful occupation, extreme physical exercise, and overzealous dietary management in order to maintain a particular desired physical appearance. Making lifestyle modifications is the important aspect of management. Patients have biochemical features of hypogonadotrophic hypogonadism and structural pituitary/hypothalamic lesions should be ruled out. Progestin challenge test if done shows minimal spotting or no withdrawal bleeding at all. It demonstrates the absence of oestrogen priming in this situation. Painful sexual intercourse, vaginal dryness may be accompanying symptoms that are, again, due to loss of oestrogen effect on vaginal mucosa. The combined oral contraceptive pill should be offered to negate the effects of low oestrogen in patients who do not respond to conservative management.

Endometrial carcinoma may be seen in patients with an unopposed oestrogen effect on endometrium, rather than in patients with hypogonadotrophic hypogonadism.

Gordon C. Functional hypothalamic amenorrhea. New England Journal of Medicine, 2010; 363: 365–371.

21. D. The combination of irregular periods, and clinical and biochemical hyper-androgenism is suggestive of a diagnosis of PCOS. Oral contraceptive pills (OCP) with ethinyl oestradiol (30–35μg) and low-dose progesterone is the first-line treatment for menstrual irregularities. The aim is to regularize her periods and reduce androgen excess. The oestrogens lead to an increase in SHBG levels resulting in a reduction of free testosterone levels. Reduction in androgen levels will result in reducing the thickness of facial/body hair. In women who fail to respond to the OCPs and have moderate to severe hirsutism, anti-androgen therapy, such as cyproterone acetate or spironolactone, can be used. Eflornithine is a topical agent used for mild hirsutism and has no impact on the menstrual irregularity. It is an ornithine decarboxylase enzyme inhibitor, which coverts ornithine to putrescine, which helps in cell division of hair follicles.

Polycystic ovarian syndrome: Clinical knowledge summaries (CKS). NICE, 2013. Available at: http://cks.nice.org.uk/polycystic-ovary-syndrome

22. D. DMPA is a progestin-only preparation, which is used once every 3 months as a deep IM preparation.

Indications:

- At least 1 year of birth spacing desired.
- Highly effective long-acting contraception not linked to coitus.
- Coitally-independent method desired.
- Need for oestrogen-free contraception.
- Breastfeeding.
- Sickle cell disease.
- Seizure disorder.

Contraindications:

Absolute

- Pregnancy.
- Un-explained genital bleeding.
- Severe coagulation disorders.
- Previous sex steroid–induced liver adenoma.

Relative

- Liver disease.
- Severe cardiovascular disease.
- Rapid return to fertility desired.
- Difficulty with injections.
- Severe depression.

Compliance is usually poor: 25% withdraw after 1 year, 50% after 2 years and up to 80% after 3 years.

23. B. This woman is in the climacteric stage, which is also known as the peri-menopausal state. The inhibin levels starts to decline after 30 years of age and this process contributes to a progressive increase in levels of FSH. The exposure of follicular cells to high FSH concentration leads to raised oestradiol levels during this period. Oestradiol levels start to fall about a year before the menopause. The peri-menopausal period is generally considered an ideal time to educate women regarding the impending menopause, and to evaluate the risks and benefits of long-term hormone replacement therapy (HRT).

Anderson R. Predicting the menopause: The role of inhibin B. Trends in Urology Gynaecology & Sexual Health, 2007; 12 (2): 9–10.

24. D. Male infertility may be due to:

- Being idiopathic 50%.
- Seminiferous tubule dysgenesis (Klinefelter's syndrome) 20%.
- Genital tract obstruction.
- Hypogonadotrophic hypogonadism (pituitary adenoma, Kallmann syndrome).
- Varicocele 15–30%.
- Miscellaneous (anti-sperm antibodies, drugs, trauma, mumps orchitis).

Causes of primary gonadal failure include:

- Klinefelter's syndrome.
- Mumps orchitis.
- Trauma.
- Iatrogenic (post-irradiation).
- Haemochromatosis.

Swerdloff RS and Wang C. Causes of male infertility. UpToDate. Available at: http://www.uptodate.com/contents/causes-of-male-infertility

25. E. Testosterone replacement therapy forms the cornerstone of the management of patients with Klinefelter's syndrome. It normally should be started during puberty and the dose increased gradually to maintain age-specific testosterone and LH levels.

26. C. The tall stature with gynaecomastia and small firm testicles, in combination with the biochemistry suggestive of primary testicular failure, are features of Klinefelter's syndrome. It is a common condition seen in 1:1000 males. The abnormality is an extra X chromosome and polysomy of X chromosome can occur. The greater the number of X chromosomes, the higher the somatic and psychological dysfunction. The seminiferous tubules undergo extensive fibrosis and hyalinization in an accelerated phase in puberty, leading to low testosterone and androgen-deficient state. In the absence of the feedback to gonadotropin s, FSH and LH are significantly elevated. There is an increased risk of breast carcinoma, aortic valvular disease, mitral valve prolapse (in 50%), bronchitis, emphysema, osteoporosis, pulmonary embolism, and berry aneurysm with this condition.

Groth K, Skakkebæk G, Høst C, et al. Clinical review: Klinefelter syndrome—a clinical update. Journal of Clinical Endocrinology & Metabolism, 2013; 98(1): 20–30.

27. C. This patient has clinical and biochemical features consistent with primary gonadal failure probably secondary to mumps orchitis. He will require testosterone replacement therapy for symptomatic improvement and to prevent osteoporosis. The management of infertility in primary hypogonadism usually requires IVF or intra-cytoplasmic sperm injection (ICSI).

Masarani M, Wazait H, and Dinneen M. Mumps orchitis. Journal of the Royal Society of Medicine 2006; 99: 573–575.

Kobayashi H, Nagao K, and Nakajima K. Focus Issue on Male Infertility. Advances in Urology, 2012; 2012: 823582.

28. D. The luteal phase of menstrual cycle is characterized by LH and FSH from the pituitary gland causing the transformation of remaining part of the dominant follicle to corpus luteum, which secretes progesterone. See Table 5.7.

Table 5.7 Physiological changes during menstrual cycle

	Follicular phase (day 1–12)	Ovulation (day 13–15)	Luteal phase (day 15–28)
Anterior pituitary	FSH>LH	LH surge	Gradual fall in LH and an increase in FSH levels
Ovary	High oestradiol as follicles mature	Ovulation	Corpus luteum formation Progesterone increase

Barrett K, Barman S, Boitano S, et al. Ganong review of physiology (24th edn), Lange Basic Science. Lange, 2012.

29 A. Androgen-secreting tumour should be suspected in the presence of any of the following clinical features:

- Rapidly progressive hirsutism.
- Very high androgen levels.
- Adrenal mass >4 cm in size.

A CT abdomen and pelvis should be organized to rule out presence of any ovarian/adrenal mass.

d'Alva C, Abiven-Lepage G, Viallon V, et al. Sex steroids in androgen-secreting adrenocortical tumors: clinical and hormonal features in comparison with non-tumoral causes of androgen excess. European Journal of Endocrinology. 2008; 159: 641–647.

30. A. Drugs that can potentially lead to hirsutism include:

- Phenytoin.
- Androgens.
- Cyclosporine.
- Danazol.
- Minoxidil.

31. E. Biochemical changes that may be seen in patients with polycystic ovarian syndrome include:

- Reversal of FSH to LH ratio.
- Low SHBG levels.
- Raised free testosterone levels.
- Raised androstenedione and DHEAS levels.

Melmed S, Polonsky K, Reed Larsen P, et al. Williams textbook of endocrinology (12th edn). Elsevier, 2011.

32. E. Anti-androgens, such as spironolactone and flutamide, can be used for the management of hirsutism that is not responding to mechanical measures (waxing, shaving, etc.) in patients with PCOS. These agents are generally avoided in patients desiring fertility due to their potential teratogenic side effects.

33. B. Patients with Klinefelter's syndrome are at an increased risk of breast cancer, non-Hodgkin's lymphoma, and lung cancer. Periodic breast examination and mammography for breast cancer surveillance is recommended for men with Klinefelter's syndrome.

Swerdlow A, Schoemaker M, Higgins C, et al. Cancer incidence and mortality in men with Klinefelter syndrome: a cohort study. Journal of the National Cancer Institute. 2005; 97(16): 1204–1210.

34. C. Long-term androgen and anabolic steroids for body building and to enhance athletic performance can potentially suppress the endogenous pituitary–gonadal axis. These individuals may present with erectile dysfunction and loss of libido, with biochemical features of hypogonadotrophic hypogonadism. The key step is to stop the use of these performance-enhancing drugs and repeat the biochemical profile in few weeks or months, although the recovery of the pituitary–gonadal axis may take months. Other potential side effects of these agents include raised LDL-cholesterol levels, deranged liver function test, hepatic neoplasm, and breast tenderness/swelling.

Rahnema C, Lipshultz L, Crosnoe E, et al. Anabolic steroid-induced hypogonadism: diagnosis and treatment. Fertility and Sterility, 2014; 101(5): 1271–1279.

35. D. NCCAH should be considered as a differential diagnosis in women labelled as PCOS who present with features of hirsutism, acne, and menstrual irregularities. A random measurement of 17-hydroxy progesterone (17-OHP) levels may be within the normal range in patients with NCCAH. A short synacthen test with measurement of 17OHP is considered the gold standard for the diagnosis of NCCAH.

36. D. Non-classic CAH is an important differential diagnosis to be considered in women presenting with features suggestive of polycystic ovarian disease (PCOS) such as menstrual irregularities and hyper-androgenism (acne, hirsutism). It is caused by a deficiency of 21 hydroxylase enzyme leading to an inadequate cortisol and aldosterone production. This results in precursors such as 17-OHP to be diverted to androgen-producing pathways, leading to hyper-androgenism. The 17-OHP levels of 5–15 nmol/L are associated with non-classic CAH. On stimulation with ACTH, a rise in 17-OHP levels over 30–45 nmol/L is suggestive of the diagnosis of non-classic CAH. The management of this condition involves prednisolone (2.5–5 mg/day) for menstrual irregularities and anti-androgens, such as cyproterone acetate for hirsutism and acne.

Gardner D and Shoback D. Greenspan's basic and clinical endocrinology (9th edn). McGraw-Hill Medical, 2011.

37. A. Prenatal testing and diagnosis will determine the successful outcome of pregnancy in patients with CAH. Ascertaining the genotype of foetus with chorionic villous sampling is the most important step, which will influence the immediate management plan. If the sex of the foetus is female, early treatment with dexamethasone (20 μg/kg of maternal weight in three divided doses) may help prevent virilization of foetus and associated complications (reconstruction surgery, gender reassignment, etc.). If the sex of the foetus is male, dexamethasone treatment is not required. Steroid therapy is also usually not required for pregnant patients with non-classic CAH.

38. D. ICSI is a procedure in which a single sperm is injected into an egg to fertilize it in vitro. The fertilized egg is subsequently transferred to the uterus for implantation.

The indications for ICSI are:

1. Low count, but normal sperm morphology.
2. Poor motility.
3. Previous vasectomy.
4. Retrograde ejaculation contributing to low sperm count.

Varghese A, Goldberg E, and Agarwal A. Current and future perspectives on intracytoplasmic sperm injection: a critical commentary. Reproductive BioMedicine Online. 2007; 15(6): 719–727.

39. B. Prostate and breast carcinoma are absolute contraindications to testosterone replacement. Benign prostate hyperplasia, polycythaemia, and sleep apnoea are relative contraindications to testosterone therapy.

Testosterone replacement should be started after detailed physical examination, including prostate and breast examination in men aged >45 years. Prostate specific antigen (PSA) and haematocrit should be checked at baseline. The baseline PSA may be low in hypogonadal men on initiation of therapy, although it can potentially increase while patients are on adequate testosterone replacement therapy.

McGill J, Shoskes D, and Sabanegh E. Androgen deficiency in older men: Indications, advantages, and pitfalls of testosterone replacement therapy. Cleveland Clinic Journal of Medicine November 2012; 79(11): 797–806.

40. E. Aromatase enzyme is involved in the conversion of testosterone to oestradiol and located in adipocytes, and brain and vascular endothelium. Increased aromatase activity in obesity leads to raised oestradiol levels, which may result in clinical and biochemical features of hypogonado-trophic hypogonadism due to negative feedback to the hypothalmo–pituitary–gonadal (HPG) axis. Increased visceral adipose tissue is also associated with increased release of cytokines and leads to a pro-inflammatory state, contributing to higher vascular risk. Weight loss has the key role in the management of such patients.

41. D. A sperm count of <15 million/mL is considered as oligospermia; it is associated with reduced rate of fertility (see Table 5.8).

Table 5.8 Summary of normal/abnormal semen analysis results

Semen analysis	Normal	Abnormal results
Quantity	2–7 mL	
Sperm count	>20 million/mL	Oligospermia <15 million
		Azoospermia: no spermatozoa in the ejaculate
Motility	≥50%	
Morphology	>30% of normal forms	Teratospermia: <30% spermatozoa with normal morphology

Agarwal A and Said T. Interpretation of basic semen analysis and advanced semen testing. In: E.S. Sabanegh (ed.) Current Clinical Urology: Male Infertility: Problems and Solutions. Humana Press, 2011: 15–22.

42. C. According to the Rotterdam criteria, the diagnosis of PCOS is based on the presence of two out of three of the following features:

- The presence of menstrual irregularities.
- Clinical and/or biochemical features of hyper-androgenism.
- Ultrasound findings of polycystic ovaries such as:
  - Bilaterally enlarged ovaries with multiple small follicles (seen in about 50%)
  - Increased ovarian size (> 10 cc)
  - 12 or more follicles measuring 2–9 mm
  - Peripheral follicles may have a string of pearl appearance
  - Hypo-echoic ovary without individual cysts (may be seen in about 25%)

The presence of ovarian cysts on ultrasound of the pelvis is not a prerequisite for the diagnosis. The exact pathogenesis of this syndrome is yet not clear, although ovarian steroidogenesis dysfunction, imbalance in pituitary/hypothalamic hormone secretion (LH/FSH imbalance), and/or insulin resistance are believed to play a part in the development of this heterogeneous syndrome.

Lujan M, Jarrett B, Brooks E, et al. Updated ultrasound criteria for polycystic ovary syndrome: reliable thresholds for elevated follicle population and ovarian volume. Human Reproduction, 2013; 28(5): 1361–1368.

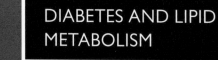

1. **DM is a global epidemic, affecting individuals in developing as well as developed countries.**

   What will be the projected prevalence of diabetes in 2030, based on estimates by the International Diabetes Federation?
   A. 50 million
   B. 360 million
   C. 550 million
   D. 1 billion
   E. 1.56 billion

2. **A 53-year-old woman presented with symptoms of increased thirst, weight loss and an increased frequency of passing urine. She had background medical history of bronchial asthma for which she occasionally used salbutamol inhaler.**

   On examination, her BMI was 29 kg/m². Her general physical and systemic examination was unremarkable except for central adiposity.

   Her fasting and random glucose readings were 6.5 and 9.2 mmol/L, respectively.

   Which one of the following biochemical cut-offs are diagnostic of diabetes, based on WHO criteria?
   A. 1-hour plasma glucose ≥11.1 on oral glucose tolerance test
   B. Fasting glucose ≥6 mmol/L, with osmotic symptoms
   C. Fasting glucose ≥7 mmol/L in an asymptomatic patient
   D. Random glucose ≥8.5 mmol/L in an asymptomatic patient
   E. Random glucose ≥11.1 mmol/L, with osmotic symptoms

3. HbA$_{1c}$ is a relatively new tool being employed for the diagnosis of
    diabetes. Although it is highly specific for the diagnosis of diabetes, it is
    not particularly sensitive, with relatively more probability of obtaining a
    false negative test result.

    Which one of the following is an appropriate indication for the use of
    HbA1c for the diagnosis of diabetes?

    A. Children
    B. Maturity onset diabetes of adulthood
    C. Patients on steroids
    D. Patients with acute pancreatic damage
    E. Pregnancy

4. A 38-year-old man of Afro-Caribbean origin presented to the medical
    assessment unit with 2-day history of feeling nauseous and generally
    unwell. He had a strong family history of diabetes. On examination, he
    had a BMI of 29 kg/m², with features of dehydration, a pulse rate of
    104 beats/minute, and blood pressure of 90 mmHg systolic. His systemic
    examination was unremarkable.

    ```
    Investigations:
      blood sugar  28 mmol/L
      pH           7.37 (7.35-7.45)
      HCO3         23 mmol/L (22-27)
      Na           134 mmol/L (135-145)
      K            4.5 mmol/L (3.5-4.5)
      amylase      22 IU/L (<125)
      urine        sugar +++, ketones 4+
    ```

    He was initially managed on a basis of insulin and intravenous fluids. He
    made a good clinical recovery and was discharged home with pre-mix
    insulin (70/30) injections bd. His subsequent blood tests show a negative
    anti-glutamic acid decarboxylase (GAD) antibody status.

    Which one of the following is the most appropriate management
    approach for him when he is reviewed on a follow-up clinic visit in
    4 weeks time?

    A. Consideration for insulin pump therapy
    B. Continue insulin therapy life long
    C. Switch to metformin
    D. Switch to pioglitazone
    E. Switch to sulfonylureas

5. **A 32-year-old woman presented to her GP with osmotic symptoms (polydipsia and polyuria). She had a background history of sensorineural deafness, with a strong family history of diabetes (mother, maternal grandmother, and few maternal cousins having type 1 or type 2 diabetes). On examination, she had a BMI of 22 kg/m², with no clinical features of Cushing's syndrome or hirsutism.**

    ```
    Investigations:
       Blood sugar   15.5 mmol/L
       pH            7.37 (7.35-7.45)
       Venous HCO3   23 mmol/L (22-27)
       Sodium        138 mmol/L (135-145)
       Potassium     4.2 mmol/L (3.5-4.5)
    ```

    Which one of the following is the most appropriate initial therapy, based on her clinical profile?

    A. Incretins

    B. Insulin

    C. Metformin

    D. Pioglitazone

    E. Sulfonylurea

6. **Which one of the following specific membrane glucose transporter is present in the highest concentration in pancreatic beta cells?**

    A. GLUT 1

    B. GLUT 2

    C. GLUT 4

    D. GLUT 5

    E. Sodium-dependent glucose transporter

7. **A 26-year-old Caucasian man with a background history of type 1 DM is keen to know the risk of his offspring developing diabetes. His wife does not have diabetes or pre-diabetes.**

    What is the risk of developing type 1 DM for a baby born to a father with type 1 DM?

    A. <1%

    B. 1–2%

    C. 3–5%

    D. 10%

    E. 25%

8. A 34-year-old woman presented to her primary care physician with osmotic symptoms such as polydipsia and polyuria. On examination, she had **BMI of 32 kg/m²** with no phenotypic features of Cushing's syndrome. Her fasting blood glucose readings are in the range 8–9 mmol/L. She is keen to know the risk of the development of type2 DM in her twin sister.

    What is the concordance rate of developing type 2 DM in monozygotic twins?

    A. <5%
    B. 5–10%
    C. 25%
    D. 30–50%
    E. 60–100%

9. As part of a research trial, a healthy medical student is detected to have islet cell (ICA), GAD, and tyrosine phosphatase-related islet antigen 2 (anti-IA-2) antibodies in her blood.

    What is the probability of developing type 1 DM in next 10 years on incidental detection of these three antibodies in the blood?

    A. <10%
    B. 15–25%
    C. 50–60%
    D. 80–90%
    E. ≥99%

10. A 40-year-old school teacher presented to the medical assessment unit with a 2-month history of osmotic symptoms and elevated blood glucose levels. There was no family history of diabetes and she was not currently on any medication. On examination, her BMI was 22 kg/m² with normal general physical and systemic examination.

    ```
    Investigations:
        random blood sugar    16.5 mmol/L
        pH                    7.40 (7.35-7.45)
        HCO3                  25 mmol/L (22-27)
        Na                    140 mmol/L (135-145)
        K                     3.7 mmol/L (3.5-4.5)
        urine                 sugar ++ Ketones - negative
    ```

    Which one of the following test may be useful in establishing the underlying diagnosis considering her clinical profile?

    A. Anti-GAD antibody
    B. Mitochondrial gene mutation (A3243G)
    C. Oral glucose tolerance test
    D. Serum ferritin and total iron binding capacity
    E. Toxicology screen

11. **A neonate aged 6 weeks presented to the paediatric emergency unit with failure to thrive and dehydration. His blood tests showed elevated blood glucose levels with low serum bicarbonate and elevated ketones, consistent with a diagnosis of diabetic ketoacidosis.**

    Which one of the following genetic mutation is associated with development of neonatal diabetes?

    A. Anti-islet cell antibodies
    B. Hepatocyte nuclear factor (HNF)-1α
    C. HNF-4β
    D. IPF-1
    E. KIR 6.2

12. **An 18-year-old boy was incidentally detected to have high fasting blood glucose readings on a routine medical check-up for army recruitment. He had no history of osmotic symptoms. He had a strong family history of diabetes with three of his first cousins and two of the paternal uncles having medication-treated diabetes. On examination, he had BMI of 23 kg/m² with normal general physical and systemic examination. His repeat blood tests confirmed elevated fasting glucose (7–9 mmol/L), although the post-prandial blood glucose was within normal range.**

    Which one of the following is the most appropriate management approach for his elevated fasting blood glucose levels?

    A. Exercise and weight loss
    B. Insulin
    C. Metformin
    D. No medications
    E. Sulphonylurea

13. **A 25-year-old man was incidentally detected to have elevated fasting as well as post-prandial blood glucose readings on routine blood tests. He had a background medical history of a renal cyst, which had been managed conservatively. He also had a strong family history of diabetes, with a few of his first cousins, uncles, and grandparents having diabetes requiring medications or insulin. On examination, he had BMI of 21 kg/m², with no peripheral stigmata of insulin resistance, such as acanthosis nigricans.**

    Which one of the following genetic mutation is most likely, based on his clinical profile?

    A. Glucokinase
    B. HNF-1α
    C. HNF-1β
    D. HNF-4 α
    E. IPF

14. A 24-year-old woman was reviewed in the diabetes clinic on a routine follow-up visit. She was diagnosed as having type 1 DM aged 16 years, when she was noted to have elevated fasting blood glucose levels on routine blood tests, while undergoing treatment for a urinary tract infection. She had been on basal-bolus insulin regimen with a total insulin requirement of 10–12 units/day. She had good glycaemic control as reflected by HbA$_{1c}$ of 46–50 mmol/mol over the last 8 years. On examination, she had a BMI of 24 kg/m^2 with no evidence of diabetic retinopathy or peripheral neuropathy.

Which one of the following characteristic feature should raise the clinical suspicion of maturity onset diabetes of the young (MODY) in this patient?

A. Absence of microvascular complications
B. Elevated fasting blood glucose
C. Good glycaemic control
D. Low insulin dose requirements
E. Multiple hypoglycaemic episodes

15. A 40-year-old man presented to his primary care physician with symptoms of polydipsia and polyuria for last 6 weeks. He had a strong family history of diabetes, with both his parents and an elder brother on oral hypoglycaemic agents or insulin for blood glucose control. On examination, he had BMI of 24 kg/m^2, with the presence of dark hyperpigmented skin in the armpit, although there was no evidence of diabetic retinopathy or peripheral neuropathy.

```
Investigations:
    random blood sugar    14.2 mmol/L
    pH                    7.43 (7.35-7.45)
    venous HCO3           24 mmol/L (22-27)
    Na                    135 mmol/L (135-145)
    K                     3.5 mmol/L (3.5-4.5)
    urine                 sugar ++ Ketones - negative
```

Which one of the following clinical/biochemical features will support the diagnosis of Type 2 DM (over a diagnosis of MODY) in this man?

A. Absence of diabetic ketoacidosis
B. Acanthosis nigricans
C. Normal BMI
D. Osmotic symptoms
E. Strong family history of diabetes

16. **A 55-year-old man was reviewed in the diabetes clinic on an annual follow-up visit. He had a background history of type 2 DM for 8 years, and taking metformin and gliclazide therapy. On examination, he had features of bilateral neuropathy.**

   Which one of the following side effects is associated with long-term metformin use?

   A. B12 deficiency
   B. Magnesium deficiency
   C. Pyridoxine deficiency
   D. Selenium deficiency
   E. Thiamine deficiency

17. **A 66-year-old woman with type 2 DM for the last 15 years presented to her primary care physician with symptoms of fatigue and weight loss. She was on metformin and sitagliptin therapy for her diabetes. On examination, she had pallor, with evidence of background diabetic retinopathy.**

   ```
   Investigations:
      Hb            12.8 g/L (12-15)
      Na            140 mmol/L (135-145)
      K             4.5 mmol/L (3.5-5.5)
      Urea          28.2 mg/dL (7-20)
      Creatinine    135 µmol/L (60-115)
      eGFR          42 mL/minute/1.73 m²
      HbA₁c         55 mmol/mol (<46)
   ```

   According to NICE guidelines, which one of the following is the correct indication to stop metformin therapy in the presence of renal impairment?

   A. eFGR <15 mL/minute/1.73 m^2
   B. eFGR <30 mL/minute/1.73 m^2
   C. eFGR <45 mL/minute/1.73 m^2
   D. eFGR <60 mL/minute/1.73 m^2
   E. eGFR <75 mL/minute/1.73 m^2

18. **Dipeptidyl peptidase inhibitors 4 (DPP4) are novel oral hypoglycaemic agents that inhibit the enzyme DPP4 and prevent breakdown of endogenous incretins.**

   Which one of the following DPP4 inhibitor is excreted unchanged in faeces and does not require any dose modification in renal disease?

   A. Alogliptin
   B. Linagliptin
   C. Saxagliptin
   D. Sitagliptin
   E. Vildagliptin

19. **Pioglitazone can be used as a second- or third-line therapy when glycaemic control remains poor, especially in presence of a significant degree of insulin resistance, although the use of this agent has been associated with complications such as congestive cardiac failure.**

    All of the following complications are associated with pioglitazone use except?

    A. Increased risk of bladder cancer
    B. Increased risk of fractures
    C. Liver toxicity
    D. Macular oedema
    E. Renal impairment

20. **Statins are the commonest agents used to manage dyslipidaemia in patients with diabetes although these have been associated with an increase risk of development of diabetes.**

    Which one of the following statins has been associated with a reduction in risk of development of DM?

    A. Atorvastatin
    B. Pitavastatin
    C. Pravastatin
    D. Rosuvastatin
    E. Simvastatin

21. **Statin therapy is the mainstay of treatment for patients with familial (homozygous or heterozygous) hypercholesterolaemia, with mixed dyslipidaemias.**

    Which one of the following biological changes is associated with use of statin therapy?

    A. Down-regulation of LDL receptors
    B. Impaired endothelial function
    C. Increase in LDL cholesterol
    D. Reduction in HDL cholesterol
    E. Up-regulation of PCSK9 expression

22. **Use of all of the following medications is believed to be associated with an adverse impact on glycaemic control except?**

    A. Atorvastatin
    B. Bisoprolol
    C. Nicotinic acid
    D. Olanzapine
    E. Protease inhibitors

23. **A 45-year-old type 2 DM man was referred to the diabetes clinic in view of his poor glycaemic control, despite being on metformin and gliclazide therapy. He had background medical history of osteoarthritis, dyslipidaemia, and hypertension. On examination, he had a BMI of 35 kg/m², with evidence of pre-proliferative diabetic retinopathy. He was considered for initiation of glucagon-like peptide (GLP-1) analogue therapy in view of his poor glycaemic control.**

    Which one of the following is a correct statement regarding GLP-1 analogue therapy use?

    A. Exenatide therapy contra-indicated if eGFR< 50 mL/minute/1.73 m²
    B. GLP-1 analogues should not be used, with insulin therapy
    C. There is increased risk of hypoglycaemia with GLP-1 analogues
    D. Need to discontinue if there is <5% body weight loss at 6 months
    E. Need to discontinue therapy if there is HbA_{1c} <1% drop at 6 months

24. **Dapagliflozin is a sodium-glucose co-transporter 2 (SGLT2) inhibitors, which has been approved by NICE to be used as second-line agent with metformin in patients with type 2 DM.**

    Which one of the following is a contraindication for use of dapagliflozin therapy?

    A. Combination with GLP-1 analogue
    B. Combination with insulin
    C. Combination with thiazides
    D. Cranial diabetes insipidus
    E. eGFR < 60 mL/minute/1.73 m²

25. **Gluconeogenesis is a process of generation of glucose from non-glucose source, such as amino-acids, glycerol, fatty acids, and lactate.**

    Which one of the following organs participate in the process of gluconeogenesis in human beings?

    A. Liver and adipose tissue
    B. Liver and kidney
    C. Liver and pancreas
    D. Pancreas and adipose tissue
    E. Pancreas and muscles

26. A 55-year-old man was reviewed in the diabetes clinic on an annual follow-up visit. He had a background history of type 2 DM for the previous 5 years, morbid obesity, and dyslipidaemia. He was a non-smoker with an alcohol intake of about 3–4 units/week. On examination, he had central obesity with a BMI of 42 kg/m².

```
Investigations:
    albumin      34 g/L (30-50)
    ALP          255 U/L (50-125)
    ALT          82 mU/L (05-58)
    bilirubin    1.2 mg/L (0.1-1)
    HbA1c        95 mmol/mol (<46)
```

His hepatitis screen, iron studies, and autoimmune screen were normal. Ultrasound of the abdomen showed fatty liver with a normal gall bladder and bile duct.

Based on his clinical profile, with the results of biochemical and radiological tests, a diagnosis of non-alcoholic fatty liver disease (NAFLD) secondary to diabetes/metabolic syndrome is considered.

Which one of the following is the cornerstone of management of patients with NAFLD?

A. Avoidance of metformin
B. Early use of insulin
C. Incretins
D. Sulfonylureas
E. Weight loss and life style measures

27. A 60-year-old man with newly-diagnosed type 2 DM presented to the diabetes clinic with symptoms of low libido, fatigue, and malaise. He also complained of non-specific abdominal pain, with stiffness of the joints. He was a non-smoker and drank 1–2 units of alcohol on weekly basis. On examination, he had a BMI of 24 kg/m², with no evidence of peripheral neuropathy or diabetic retinopathy.

```
Investigations:
    albumin                  30 g/L (30-50)
    ALP                      205 U/L (50-125)
    ALT                      115 mU/L (05-58)
    bilirubin                1.9 mg/L (0.1-1)
    HbA1c                    71 mmol/mol (<46)
    ferritin                 450 pmol/L (10-300)
    transferrin saturation   50%
```

Which one of the following is the probable diagnosis, based on his clinical profile?

A. Glycogen storage disease
B. Haemochromatosis
C. Maturity onset diabetes of adulthood
D. Mitochondrial disease
E. Pancreatic carcinoma

28. **A 33-year-old Caucasian woman was reviewed on a routine antenatal check-up when she was 16 week pregnant.**

   According to NICE guidelines for the management of diabetes in pregnancy, the presence of all of the following factors should act as a trigger to screen for gestational diabetes except?
   A. Body mass index >25 kg/m^2
   B. Family history of diabetes (first degree relatives)
   C. Previous gestational diabetes
   D. Previous macrosomic baby (weighing >4.5 kg)
   E. South East Asian ethnic origin

29. **A 26-year-old woman with type 1 DM was reviewed in the diabetes clinic on a routine visit. She was currently on a basal-bolus insulin regimen, with good glycaemic control as evidenced by a HbA$_{1c}$ value of 48 mmol/mol. She was keen to start a family and sought pre-conception advice.**

   According to NICE guidelines, all of the following are correct regarding management of patients with diabetes in the preconception period except?
   A. Folic acid supplement
   B. Monthly HbA$_{1c}$ measurement
   C. Renal referral if eGR < 60 mL/minute/1.73 m^2
   D. Retinal screening (if not done in last 1 year)
   E. Stop statins

30. **A 24-year-old woman with type 1 DM, diagnosed 6 years ago, was reviewed during a routine follow-up visit to the antenatal clinic. She was taking a basal-bolus insulin regimen and had a sub-optimal preconception glycaemic control as reflected by a HbA$_{1c}$ of 62 mmol/mol. She was keen to assess the risk of congenital malformation in her offspring.**

   What is the relative risk of developing congenital malformations in children born to mothers with diabetes compared with the non-diabetic population?
   A. No increased risk
   B. 1.5–2-fold increased risk
   C. 4–5-fold increased risk
   D. 7–8-fold increased risk
   E. >10-fold increased risk

31. **A 25-year-old Caucasian school teacher with type 1 DM was reviewed in the joint antenatal–diabetes clinic when she was 12 weeks pregnant.**

    All of the following factors are associated with an adverse pregnancy outcome in a patient with diabetes except?

    A. Ethnic origin
    B. Poor preconception glycaemic control
    C. Preconception diabetic complications
    D. Smoking
    E. Socio-economic status

32. **A 28-year-old woman with type 1 DM for previous 16 years presented to the joint antenatal–diabetes clinic on a routine follow-up visit. She was on a basal-bolus insulin regimen with a satisfactory glycaemic control (HbA$_{1c}$ 48 mmol/mol, preconception).**

    According to NICE guidelines, which one of the following is the correct statement for blood glucose monitoring in pregnancy for women with diabetes?

    A. Aim for a fasting blood glucose level 4.5–6.5 mmol/L
    B. Aim for a 2-hour post-prandial glucose level <8 mmol/L
    C. HbA$_1$c <46 mmol/mol in the third trimester
    D. Individualized targets for monitoring
    E. Measure fasting and 2-hour post-prandial blood glucose levels

33. **A 37-year-old lady with type 2 DM was reviewed in diabetes clinic on a routine follow-up visit. She was on metformin and ramipril therapy with a good glycaemic control as reflected by a HbA$_{1c}$ of 50 mmol/mol. She was keen to start a family and seeks pre-conception advice.**

    According to NICE guidelines, which one of the following is the correct statement regarding her further management during pregnancy?

    A. Aspart and lispro insulin are contraindicated
    B. Continue ramipril
    C. Isophane insulin can be used if required
    D. Start atorvastatin
    E. Stop metformin

34. **A 36-year-old woman with type 2 DM was reviewed on a routine follow-up visit to the diabetes clinic. She was planning to start a family and keen to assess the risk of development of congenital malformations and perinatal mortality in her offspring.**

    Which one of the following statements is correct regarding the risk of perinatal mortality and congenital malformations in the offspring of women with type 2 diabetes, compared with women with type 1 diabetes?

    A. 1.5–2-fold less risk

    B. 4–5-fold less risk

    C. 1.5–2-fold increased risk

    D. 4–5-fold increased risk

    E. Same risk as women with type 1 diabetes

35. **Which one of the following is the correct diagnostic criterion for the diagnosis of gestational diabetes for the 75 g OGTT based on International Association of Diabetes and Pregnancy Study Groups (IADPSG) report published in 2010?**

    A. Fasting >5.1 mmol/L

    B. Fasting >7 mmol/L

    C. 1-hour value >7.8 mmol/L

    D. 2-hour value >7.8 mmol/L

    E. 2-hour value >10 mmol/L

36. **A 45-year-old man of Afro-Caribbean origin is reviewed in the diabetes clinic on a routine follow-up visit. He had a background history of type 2 DM, hypertension, and sickle cell disease. He was injecting isophane insulin bd, with metformin sustained-release tablets. His home blood glucose monitoring readings were variable with a range of 10–15 mmol/L throughout the day. He had not suffered from any hypoglycaemic episode in recent months.**

    Which one of the following is the most accurate parameter to assess his glycaemic control?

    A. Fasting glucose

    B. Fructosamine

    C. Glucosamine HbA_{1c}

    D. HbA_{1c}

    E. Oral glucose tolerance test

37. **A 55-year-old man of South East Asian origin presented to his general practitioner with a 2-month history of weight loss and increased thirst. He had a family history of thalassemia D. He was on doxazosin and ramipril tablets for blood pressure control.**

    On examination, his BMI was 28 kg/m². His general physical and systemic examination was unremarkable.

    ```
    Investigations:
      Hb                  9.6 g/L (12-15)
      urea                24.5 mg/dL (7-20)
      creatinine          130 µmol/L (60-115)
      eGFR                55 mL/minute/1.73 m²
      HbA1c               38 mmol/mol (<46)
      fasting glucose     9.5 mmol/L
    ```

    All of the following are associated with a false negative HbA1c results except?

    A. Doxazosin
    B. Haemoglobinopathy
    C. Haemolytic anaemia
    D. Pregnancy
    E. Renal impairment

38. **A 63-year-old man with type 2 DM was reviewed during his routine follow-up visit to the clinic. He was on metformin, gliclazide, and ramipril tablets. On examination, he had a BMI of 28 kg/m² with central obesity.**

    ```
    Investigations:
      Albumin             35 g/L (30-50)
      ALP                 115 U/L (50-125)
      ALT                 35 mU/L (05-58)
      bilirubin           0.5 mg/L (0.1-1)
      HbA1c               50 mmol/mol (<46)
      triglycerides       3.5 mmol/L
      LDL cholesterol     3.2 mmol/L
    ```

    Which one of the following is the most appropriate next step for the further management of his elevated triglyceride levels?

    A. Check TFT and renal function
    B. Repeat triglyceride levels in 3 months
    C. Start fibrates
    D. Start omega fatty acids
    E. Start statins

39. **A 62-year-old retired school teacher attended the diabetes clinic on a routine follow-up visit. He had undergone bariatric surgery for his morbid obesity associated with type 2 DM and obstructive sleep apnoea about 6 months previously. He had noticed a significant amount of weight loss during this period, although he complained of visual symptoms that were more noticeable during late evening hours.**

Deficiency of which one of the following vitamins/nutrients is the probable explanation for his visual symptoms?

A. Magnesium
B. Vitamin A
C. Vitamin B12
D. Vitamin D
E. Zinc

40. **A 55-year-old man with Type 2 DM for 15 years was reviewed in the diabetes clinic on a routine follow-up visit. He was on metformin and gliclazide tablets. On examination, he had a BMI of 27 kg/m², and a blood pressure of 145/90 mmHg, with evidence of background diabetic retinopathy.**

```
Investigations:
    LDL cholesterol              5.2 mmol/L
    triglycerides                2.6 mmol/L (<2)
    HbA₁c                        62 mmol/mol (<46)
    urine albumin creatinine ratio   25.5 mg/mmol (<2.5)
```

Which one of the following is a correct statement with regards to the presence of albuminuria in patients with diabetes?

A. ACE inhibitors are indicated only in hypertensive patients with albuminuria.
B. Albuminuria is associated with a decline in eGFR
C. Albuminuria is often due to exercise and prolonged standing
D. Albuminuria is strongly associated with presence of autonomic neuropathy
E. Urine ACR needs to be repeated at 3–6-monthly interval

41. **A 55-year-old woman was reviewed in the diabetes clinic on a routine follow-up appointment. She had poorly-controlled type 2 diabetes (for the previous 8 years), with history of dyslipidaemia, osteoarthritis, obstructive sleep apnoea, and depression. She was mostly housebound and felt anxious about venturing out due to poor self-image leading to suicidal ideation for which she is under psychiatry review. On examination, she had a BMI of 45 kg/m², with central obesity.**

Which one of the following is the most appropriate step in her further management?

A. Bariatric surgery
B. GLP-1 analogue
C. Insulin
D. Orlistat
E. SGLT2 inhibitors

42. **A 19-year-old university student with type 1 diabetes mellitus was reviewed in the adolescent diabetes clinic. She had been on meal time aspart insulin injections (tds, dose based on carbohydrate counting), with a basal injection of glargine insulin at night-time. Her home blood glucose readings were variable ranging from 5 to 15 mmol/L and her HbA₁c readings were 75 mmol/mol (9%).**

   According to NICE guidelines (July 2008), which one of the following is the correct HbA₁c cut-off recommended for the use of continuous subcutaneous insulin infusion (insulin pump) in adults and children over age >12 years with type 1 DM?

   A. 8.0%
   B. 8.5%
   C. $\geq$9.0%
   D. $\geq$9.5%
   E. $\geq$10%

43. **A 65-year-old man presented to medical assessment unit with generalized lethargy, nausea, and malaise. He had a background history of type 2 DM and end-stage renal failure, and was waiting to begin haemodialysis therapy. He was oliguric on admission.**

   On examination, he was clinically dehydrated, his blood pressure was 150/60 mmHg, and he had a pulse rate of 70 beats/minute. His systemic examination was unremarkable.

   ```
   Investigations:
     Na                    106 mmol/L (135-145)
     K                     6.0 mmol/L (3.5-5.5)
     urea                  30 mg/dL (5-9)
     creatinine            565 µmol/L (60-115)
     free T4               15.5 pmol/L (0.9-19.1)
     TSH                   0.55 mU/L (0.35-5.00)
     serum osmolality      292 mOsmol/kg (275-295)
     urine osmolality      502 mOsmol/kg
     urine sodium          <20 mmol/L
   ```

   Which one of the following is the correct management approach for this patient?

   A. Fluid restriction
   B. Hydrocortisone (intravenous/intramuscular)
   C. Intravenous fluids and insulin infusion
   D. Intravenous fluids only
   E. Prednisolone (orally)

44. **A 70-year-old woman presented with sudden-onset headache and nausea. She had a background history of hypertension, osteoarthritis, and dyslipidaemia. She was taking amlodipine, atorvastatin, and paracetamol tablets. On examination, she had an elevated blood pressure of 190/104 mmHg, a Glasgow coma score (GCS) of 15/15 with normal systemic examination and no focal neurological deficit.**

```
Investigations:
    Na                  128 mmol/L (135-145)
    K                   5.2 mmol/L (3.5-5.5)
    urea                10 mg/dL (5-9)
    creatinine          125 µmol/L (60-115)
    free T4             7.5 pmol/L (0.9-19.1)
    TSH                 0.17 mU/L (0.35-5.00)
    serum osmolality    280 mOsmol/kg (275-295)
    urine osmolality    442 mOsmol/kg
    Urine sodium        42 mmol/L
```

Which one of the following is the most appropriate next step in her management?

A. CT pituitary

B. Fluid restriction

C. Thyroid uptake scan

D. Tolvaptan

E. 3% normal saline

45. An 88-year-old man presented to the medical assessment unit with a history of recurrent falls and increasing confusion. He had a background history of vascular dementia, previous stroke, and dyslipidaemia. He was currently on ramipril, phenytoin, simvastatin, frusemide, and aspirin therapy.

On examination, his blood pressure was 104/70 mmHg, he had a pulse of 94 beats/minute, and normal systemic examination, with no focal neurological deficit.

```
Investigations:
  Na                    121 mmol/L (135-145)
  K                     3.2 mmol/L (3.5-5.5)
  urea                  12.8 mg/dL (5-9)
  creatinine            91 µmol/L (60-115)
  free T4               14.4 pmol/L (0.9-19.1)
  TSH                   8.1 mU/L (0.35-5.00)
  serum osmolality      263 mOsmol/kg (275-295)
  urine osmolality      360 mOsmol/kg
  urine sodium          40 mmol/L
  random cortisol       502 nmol/L
```

Which one of the following is the most appropriate management approach in his case?

A. Demeclocycline

B. Fluid restriction

C. Hydrocortisone

D. Saline infusion

E. 3% saline

46. **A 62-year-old woman presented with increasing drowsiness and developed atonic clonic seizure while she was in the medical assessment unit. She had a background history of hypertension and osteoporosis. She was currently on amlodipine and alendronate therapy. On examination, she was well hydrated, with normal systemic examination. There was no focal neurological deficit.**

```
Investigations:
    Na                  117 mmol/L (135-145)
    K                   4.0 mmol/L (3.5-5.5)
    urea                6.8 mg/dL (5-9)
    creatinine          101 µmol/L (60-115)
    free T4             12.5 pmol/L (0.9-19.1)
    TSH                 7.2 mU/L (0.35-5.00)
    serum osmolality    252 mOsmol/kg (275-295)
    urine osmolality    180 mOsmol/kg
    urine sodium        48 mmol/L
    random cortisol     432 nmol/L
    CT head             normal study
```

Which one of the following is the most appropriate management approach in her clinical scenario?

A. Demeclocycline

B. Fluid restriction (0.5–1 L/day)

C. Hydrocortisone

D. 0.9% Saline infusion (2 L over 24 hours)

E. 3% saline

47. **A 67-year-old retired professor was reviewed in the diabetes clinic on a routine follow-up visit. He was diagnosed as having type 2 diabetes about 8 years earlier, and was taking metformin and gliclazide tablets. He was a known patient with hypertension, currently on amlodipine and ramipril tablets. On examination, he had a BMI of 30.5 kg/m², with evidence of central adiposity. There was evidence of bilateral background diabetic retinopathy on ophthalmological examination.**

```
Investigations:
   urea                              25.5 mg/dL (7-20)
   creatinine                        145 µmol/L (60-115)
   eGFR                              42 mL/minute/1.73 m²
   HbA1c                             50 mmol/mol (<46)
   Urine albumin creatinine ratio   > 300 mg/mmol
```

Which one of the following is suggestive of an alternative aetiology for the renal impairment, rather than development of diabetic nephropathy?

A. Absence of active sediment in urine

B. Duration of type 2 DM >5 years

C. The presence of diabetic retinopathy

D. Rapid decline in eGFR

E. Systemic hypertension

48. **A 54-year-old woman was reviewed in the diabetes clinic on a routine follow-up visit. She was diagnosed to have diabetes about 5 years earlier, and was taking glimepride and sitagliptin tablets. She was a known patient, with primary biliary cirrhosis with portal hypertension and under regular gastroenterology follow-up. On examination, she had a BMI of 17.5 kg/m² with evidence of muscle wasting. She had a bilateral background diabetic retinopathy on ophthalmological examination.**

```
Investigations:
   urea                              18.0 mg/dL (7-20)
   creatinine                        108 µmol/L (60-115)
   eGFR                              62 mL/minute/1.73 m²
   HbA1c                             54 mmol/mol (<46)
   urine albumin creatinine ratio   > 300 mg/mmol
```

Which one of the following is a relatively more accurate parameter to monitor renal function in patients with diabetes who have co-existent liver cirrhosis?

A. Albumin creatinine ratio

B. Serum chromogranin B

C. Serum creatinine

D. Serum cystatin C

E. Urinary C peptide

49. **A 52-year-old man presented to the diabetes clinic with a 3-month history of excruciating pain in his feet, which was keeping him awake in the night. He was diagnosed as having type 1 diabetes in his early 20s and had been on a basal-bolus insulin regimen (short-acting human insulin with meals, with a glargine insulin injection in the evening). On examination, he had bilateral pre-proliferative diabetic retinopathy changes, with reduced vibration, as well as pin-prick sensation (as checked by monofilament) in the feet.**

```
Investigations:
   urea          22.0 mg/dL (7-20)
   creatinine    122 µmol/L (60-115)
   eGFR          68 mL/minute/1.73 m²
   HbA₁c         79 mmol/mol (<46)
```

According to NICE guidelines (CG96), which one of the following is the first-line treatment for his symptoms suggestive of painful peripheral neuropathy?

A. Amitriptyline
B. Duloxetine
C. Gabapentin
D. Pregablin
E. Tramadol

50. **A 16-year-old girl presented to her general practitioner with an 8-week history of increased thirst, weight loss, and increased frequency of micturition. She had no previous history of any medical illness. On examination, she had mild dehydration and her systemic examination was normal.**

```
Investigations:
   Na               133 mmol/L (135-145)
   K                3.6 mmol/L (3.5-5.5)
   urea             8.5 mg/dL (5-9)
   creatinine       110 µmol/L (60-115)
   random glucose   18.5 mmol/L
```

A clinical diagnosis of type 1 DM was made, based on her osmotic symptoms, with elevated blood glucose levels.

According to NICE guidelines (CG15), children and young people with type 1 diabetes should be offered screening for all of the following except?

A. Addison's disease at diagnosis
B. Blood pressure annually (from age of 12 years)
C. Coeliac disease at diagnosis
D. Thyroid disease annually
E. Thyroid disease at diagnosis

51. **A 25-year-old man of South East Asian origin was incidentally detected to have an elevated random blood glucose level of 15 mmol/L, while he underwent routine blood tests. He had no previous history of medical illness and was not on any regular medications. He had no family history of diabetes. On examination, his BMI was 26 kg/m². His general physical and systemic examination was unremarkable.**

```
Investigations:
    Na                135 mmol/L (135-145)
    K                 4.5 mmol/L (3.5-5.5)
    urea              7.5 mg/dL (5-9)
    creatinine        90 µmol/L (60-115)
    fating glucose    9.5 mmol/L
    HbA1c             103 mmol/mol (<46)
```

The presence of which one of the following clinical/biochemical feature is suggestive of a diagnosis of type 1 diabetes (as against a diagnosis of type 2 diabetes)?

A. BMI of 26

B. Grossly elevated HbA$_{1c}$ levels

C. Lack of family history

D. Presence of ketonuria

E. South East Asian ethnic origin

52. **A 54-year-old man was reviewed in the diabetes clinic on a follow-up visit. He was diagnosed as having type 2 diabetes for the previous 8 years and was on two oral hypoglycaemic agents (metformin and gliclazide). His glycaemic control was suboptimal as reflected by elevated home blood glucose readings. On examination, he had a BMI of 30 kg/m². He had bilateral background diabetic retinopathy changes in the eyes.**

```
Investigations:
    urea              10.5 mg/dL (5-9)
    creatinine        125 µmol/L (60-115)
    fating glucose    7.5 mmol/L
    eGFR              55 mL/minute/ 1.73 m²
    HbA1c             63 mmol/mol (<46)
```

Which one of the following is the most appropriate next step in his management based on NICE guidelines (CG87)?

A. DPP 4 inhibitor

B. GLP-I analogue

C. Human NPH insulin

D. Insulin degludec

E. No change required

53. **A 48-year-old man with type 1 diabetes for over three decades was reviewed in the diabetes clinic. He had been on basal-bolus insulin with a sub-optimal glycaemic control, as reflected by elevated home blood glucose readings. He had noticed a deterioration in his vision over the previous 4 weeks. On examination, he had evidence of venous loops and exudates within a disc diameter of the centre of the fovea.**

    All of the following are indications for referral to the ophthalmologist in a patient with diabetic retinopathy except?

    A. Cotton wool spots
    B. Exudates within macula
    C. Multiple blot haemorrhages
    D. Unexplained drop in visual acuity
    E. Venous beading and loops

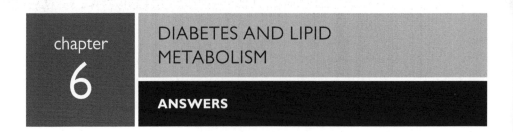

1. C. According to the international diabetes federation statistics 366 million people are currently afflicted by diabetes and the numbers will rise to 550 million by year 2030. Around 80% of patients with diabetes live in low and middle income countries, and about half of them remain undiagnosed. Diabetes affects all age group, with the maximum number of individuals falling in the age bracket 40–59 years.

International Diabetes Federation. IDF Diabetes Atlas, 6th edn. IDF, 2013. Available at: http://www.idf.org/diabetesatlas

2. E. According to the WHO criteria for the diagnosis of diabetes:

- A patient is diagnosed to have diabetes if he/she has osmotic symptoms, with biochemical evidence of:
  - random glucose ≥11.1 mmol/L; or
  - fasting glucose ≥7 mmol/L; or
  - 2-hour plasma glucose ≥11.1 on oral glucose tolerance test.
- An asymptomatic patient is diagnosed to have diabetes if he/she has biochemical evidence of a fasting glucose ≥7 mmol/L or random glucose ≥11.1, with a second confirmatory plasma venous glucose measurement, to be repeated on another day with the glucose reading in diabetic range (fasting, random, or 2-hour post-glucose tolerance test).

Data from Definition and diagnosis of diabetes mellitus and intermediate hyperglycaemia. Report of a WHO/IDF consultation. 2006. ISBN: 9789241594936.

Definition and diagnosis of diabetes mellitus and intermediate hyperglycaemia. Report of a WHO/IDF consultation. WHO, 2006.

3. B. HbA$_{1c}$ is not appropriate for use in the diagnosis of diabetes in the following situations:

- Patients on steroids or antipsychotics that can increase blood glucose readings.
- Patients with acute pancreatic damage.
- Pregnancy.
- Patients suspected to have type 1 DM.
- Children and young adults.
- Haemoglobinopathies, which can influence HbA1c results.
- Patients with short duration of osmotic symptoms.

Farmer A. Use of HbA1c in the diagnosis of diabetes. British Medical Journal, 2012; 345: e7293.

4. C. Ketosis prone diabetes is more common in black and Hispanic ethnic subgroups. The patients are generally obese and may present with features of diabetic ketoacidosis. The autoimmune antibody status (anti-GAD antibodies) is generally negative. The management is initially on the lines of diabetic ketoacidosis (fluids/insulin/potassium replacement). Most of these patients can be managed on oral hypoglycaemic agents with the discontinuation of insulin therapy within a few weeks to months.

Balasubramanyam A, Garza G, Rodriguez L, et al. Accuracy and predictive value of classification schemes for ketosis-prone diabetes. Diabetes Care, 2006; 29(12): 2575–2579.

Mauvais-Jarvis F, Sobngwi E, Porcher R, et al. Ketosis-prone type 2 diabetes in patients of sub-Saharan African origin: clinical pathophysiology and natural history of beta-cell dysfunction and insulin resistance. Diabetes. 2004; 53(3): 645–653.

5. E. Mitochondrial diabetes is suspected in female patients with a strong familial clustering of diabetes, with predominantly maternal transmission of disease and the presence of sensorineural deafness. The degree and severity of insulinopenia is variable, with patients developing either type 1 or type 2 DM. The underlying defect in the majority of patients is the mitochondrial gene mutation (A3243G). The initial treatment of individuals with type 2 DM presentation due to an underlying mitochondrial mutation can be with sulfonylureas. Metformin is contraindicated due to risk of development of lactic acidosis. Hearing defects usually precede the development of diabetes in these patients.

Maassen JA, Hart LM, Van Essen E, et al. Mitochondrial diabetes: molecular mechanisms and clinical presentation. Diabetes, 2004; 53(Suppl. 1): S103–S109.

6. B. Specific membrane transporters are involved in the transport of glucose into the cells. There are two major categories of these membrane transporters being either sodium-dependent or -independent glucose transporters. The sodium-dependent transporters absorb glucose against its concentration gradient, while the sodium-independent transporters have an insulin-responsive isoform and further subdivided into Glut 1–7. Glut 2 is expressed in highest concentration in pancreatic β cells, the basolateral membrane of intestine, renal epithelial cells, and hepatocytes. Glut 4 is expressed in highest concentration in insulin-sensitive tissue such as skeletal and cardiac muscle, with adipose tissue. Glut 5 is the only transporter that has higher specificity for fructose.

Thorens B and Mueckler M. Glucose transporters in the 21st century. American Journal of Physiology—Endocrinology and Metabolism, 2010; 298(2): E141–E145.

7. C. The risk of developing type 1 DM is around 1–2% for babies born to mothers with type 1 DM (Table 6.1). This risk increases to 3–5% if the father of the baby has type 1 DM (and mother does not have diabetes). The concordance rate of developing type 1 DM is 30–35% in monozygotic twins.

Table 6.1 Inheritance rate of type 1 and type 2 DM

	Type 1 DM	Type 2 DM
Concordance rate in monozygotic twins	35%	70–90%
Mother with diabetes	1–2% increased risk	20–30% increased risk
Father with diabetes	3–5% increased risk	20–30% increased risk

Turner H and Wass J. Oxford Handbook of Endocrinology and Diabetes (2nd edn). Oxford University Press, 2009.

Pociot F and McDermott M. Genetics of type 1 diabetes mellitus Genes and Immunity 2002; 3: 235–249.

8. E. The concordance rate of developing type 2 DM in monozygotic twins is 60–100% as compared with a 30–35% concordance rate of developing type 1 DM. This is indicative of a stronger genetic component to develop type 2 DM as compared with type 1 DM, although the human leukocyte antigen (HLA)-linked genes such as HLA-DR3-DQ2/DR4-DQ8 genotype are more strongly associated with the risk of developing later (20-fold increase of developing type1 DM as compared with the general population), rather than the former.

Turner H and Wass J. Oxford Handbook of Endocrinology and Diabetes (2nd edn). Oxford University Press, 2009.

9. D. The presence of ICA, GAD, and tyrosine phosphatase-related IA-2 antibodies in the blood of a patient without diabetes, increases the 10-year risk of development of type 1 DM to 80–90%.

Lorini R, Alibrandi A, Vitali L, et al. Risk of type 1 diabetes development in children with incidental hyperglycaemia. Diabetes Care, 2001; 24(7): 1210–1216.

Turner H and Wass J. Oxford Handbook of Endocrinology and Diabetes (2nd edn). Oxford University Press, 2009.

10. A. Latent autoimmune diabetes of adulthood is a subtype of diabetes in which patients may present with phenotypic features of type 2 DM, while displaying the presence of markers of auto-immunity (anti-GAD antibodies). Most of these patients are in the age group of 30–50 years, may or may not have a normal BMI (obesity can be a confounding factor) and may present with elevated blood glucose levels, with osmotic symptoms. These patients can be managed initially with oral hypoglycaemic agents, although the β-cell function may decline over months to a few years, necessitating a relatively early requirement for insulin use.

Nambam B, Aggarwal S, and Jain A. Latent autoimmune diabetes of adults: a distinct but heterogenous clinical entity. World J Diabetes, 2010; 1(4): 111–115.

Stenstrom G, Gottsater A, Bakhtadze E, et al. Latent autoimmune diabetes in adults. definition, prevalence, β-cell function, and treatment. Diabetes, 2005; 54(Suppl. 2): S68–S72.

11. E. Neonatal diabetes usually develops within first 6 months of birth and is associated with gene mutations such as *KCNJ11* and *ABCC8* (encoding for KIR 6.2 and SUR1 subunit of pancreatic K-ATP channel involved in insulin secretion). Treatment is with insulin and a high caloric intake initially, although the patients may be responsive to sulfonylurea therapy and a switch to sulfonylureas should be considered once clinically stable.

The following features help to distinguish monogenetic diabetes from type 1 DM in children:

- Onset within 6 months of birth (*KCNJ11* or *ABCC8* mutation).
- Milder hyperglycaemia (glucokinase mutation).
- Asymptomatic hyperglycaemia.

Gloyn A, Pearson E, Antcliff J, et al. Activating mutations in the gene encoding the ATP-sensitive potassium-channel subunit Kir6.2 and permanent neonatal diabetes. New England Journal of Medicine, 2004; 350(18): 1838–1849.

12. D. Glucokinase mutation is associated with altered glucose sensing in the pancreatic β-cells, leading to mild hyperglycaemia with elevated fasting blood glucose readings. This can be managed with diet and most individuals do not develop any microvascular complication on a long-term basis.

Diabetes Research Department and the Centre for Molecular Genetics at the University of Exeter Medical School and Royal Devon and Exeter Hospital, Exeter, UK, 2014. Available at:http://www.diabetesgenes.org (suggested further reading)

13. C. MODY usually affects 1–2% of individuals with diabetes, although most cases remain unrecognized. The characteristics of MODY include a diagnosis before the fourth decade of age, a strong family history of diabetes, and absence of surrogate markers of insulin resistance (lack of central obesity, acanthosis nigricans, dyslipidaemia).

HNF-1β mutation is characterized by an association with genitourinary malformations, such as renal cysts and uterine abnormalities.

Table 6.2 summarizes the characteristic features of various MODY disorders.

Table 6.2 Characteristic features of various MODY disorder

Type	Mutation	Prevalence (% of total patients with MODY)	Clinical features
MODY 1	HNF-4α	5–10%	Progressive β-cell decline, neonatal hyperinsulinaemia, and hypoglycaemia. Responsive to sulfonylurea
MODY 2	Glucokinase	30–70%	Usually no risk of development of microvascular complications. Mild fasting hyperglycaemia
MODY 3	HNF-1α	30–70%	Marked sensitivity to sulfonylurea therapy
MODY 4	IPF1	<1%	Onset after age>35 years, pancreatic agenesis in homozygotes
MODY 5	HNF-1β	5–10%	Associated with renal cysts, genitourinary tract malformations
Neonatal diabetes	KCNJ11 ABCC8	<1%	Present with high blood glucose values during first 6 months of life, responsive to sulfonylureas

Diabetes genes. Genetic types of diabetes including maturity-onset diabetes of the young (MODY). Diabetes Research Department and the Centre for Molecular Genetics at the University of Exeter Medical School and Royal Devon and Exeter Hospital, Exeter, UK, 2014. Available at www. diabetes genes.org

14. D. The following laboratory or clinical characteristics should raise the clinical suspicion of MODY in patients labelled as type 1 DM after 3–5 years of diagnosis:

- Persistent urinary c peptides detection.
- Low insulin dose requirement (<0.5 units/kg/day).
- No tendency to develop diabetic ketoacidosis.
- Absence of anti-GAD and ICAs.
- Strong family history of diabetes.

15. B. The following clinical characteristics should raise the clinical suspicion of MODY in patients labelled as type 2 DM:

- Younger age of onset (<45 years).
- Normal BMI.
- Strong family history of diabetes.
- Fasting hyperglycaemia with no or mildly elevated post-prandial glucose (glucokinase mutation).
- Renal cysts, genitourinary tract abnormalities (HNF-1β mutation).
- Absence of surrogate markers of insulin resistance, such as acanthosis nigricans, central obesity, dyslipidaemia, hypertension.
- Marked sensitivity to sulfonylurea therapy (HNF-1α or HNF-4α mutation).

Thanabalasingham G and Owen K. Diagnosis and management of maturity onset diabetes of the young (MODY). British Medical Journal, 2011; 343: d6044.

16. A. Metformin is the most commonly used first-line medication for the management of type 2 DM. Its use has been linked with malabsorption of vitamin B12 and intrinsic factor from ileum, which can lead to peripheral neuropathy, mental changes, and macrocytic anaemia. The B12 deficiency with metformin is progressive and routine assessment of B12 levels should be considered in patients on long term metformin therapy.

Jager J, Kooy A, Lehert P, et al. Long term treatment with metformin in patients with type 2 diabetes and risk of vitamin B-12 deficiency: randomised placebo controlled trial. British Medical Journal 2010; 340: c2181.

17. B. According to the NICE guidelines (CG87), metformin dose needs to be reviewed if serum creatinine >130 μmol/L or eGFR <45 mL/minute/1.73 m². The metformin therapy should be stopped if serum creatinine >150 μmol/L or eGFR <45 mL/minute/1.73 m².

NICE. Type 2 diabetes: the management of type 2 diabetes. Guideline CG87. NICE, 2009.

18. B. Linagliptin is a DPP4 inhibitor that is predominantly excreted unchanged in faeces with metabolism of the drug playing a minor role in overall pharmacokinetics. It is a weak inhibitor of cytochrome P450. There is no dose adjustment required for linagliptin in renal failure patients.

Heise T, Graefe-Mody E, Huttner S, et al. Pharmacokinetics, pharmacodynamics and tolerability of multiple oral doses of linagliptin, a dipeptidyl peptidase-4 inhibitor in male type 2 diabetes patients. Diabetes Obesity Metabolism, 2009; 11(8): 786–794.

Drugs.com. Linagliptin. Available at: http://www.drugs.com/ppa/linagliptin.html

19. E. Pioglitazone and rosiglitazone are thiazolidinedione compounds, which act as peroxisome proliferator-activated receptors γ-agonists and help reduce peripheral insulin resistance. There is an increased incidence of heart failure in patients on pioglitazone therapy, with the risk of fluid retention. Pioglitazone has also been linked with a small increased risk of bladder carcinoma, and should not be used in patients with risk factors for bladder cancer and unexplained haematuria. The liver function needs to be monitored for the patients on pioglitazone therapy. There are case reports linking the development of macular oedema with the use of pioglitazone therapy. This agent has also been associated with an increased risk of fractures.

Rosiglitazone use was also associated with increased cardiovascular risks and it was withdrawn from the market on 2010, following a review by European Medicines agency.

Shah P and Mudaliar S. Pioglitazone: side effects and safety profile. Expert Opinion in Drug Safety, 2010; 9(2): 347–354.

de Vries C and Russel-Jones D. Rosiglitazone or pioglitazone in type 2 diabetes. British Medical Journal, 2009; 339: b3076.

20. B. Statin use has been linked with an increased risk of the development of diabetes. A meta-analysis of five trials (PROVE-IT, A to Z, TNT, IDEAL, and SEARCH), involving more than 32,000 patients without diabetes, compared the effects of high dose statins with conventional dose statins with a 12% increased risk of developing diabetes in the former compared with the later.

In another meta-analysis of 13 statin trials, 4278 individuals out of a total of 91,140 participants, developed diabetes during a mean period of 4 years, equating to a 9% increased risk for development of diabetes while on statin therapy.

On the contrary, the sub-group analysis results of the LIVES trial (Livalo Effectiveness and Safety) have shown improvement in glucose homeostasis, with an increase in HDL-cholesterol levels with pitavastatin use.

Sattar N, Preiss D, Murray HM, et al. Statins and risk of incident diabetes: a collaborative meta-analysis of randomised statin trials. Lancet, 2010; 375(9716): 735–742.

Huupponen R and Viikari J. Editorial: Statins and the risk of developing diabetes. British Medical Journal, 2013; 346: f3156.

21. E. Statins have been the mainstay therapy to lower LDL cholesterol levels in patients with both homozygous, as well as heterozygous hypercholesterolemia, with efficacy ranging from 15% to 53%, based on agent and dose used. These agents act by inhibiting the hydroxy-3-methylglutaryl-coenzyme A reductase enzyme. Statins also lead to an up-regulation of both LDL-receptor, as well as proprotein convertase substilisin kexin 9 (PCKS9) expression. PCSK9 is a key regulator of LDL-C levels as it promotes lysosomal mediated degradation of the LDL-receptor. The up-regulation of PCSK9 expression significantly attenuates the LDL-C lowering potential of statins.

Mayne J, Dewpura T, Raymond A, et al. Plasma PCSK9 levels are significantly modified by statins and fibrates in humans. Lipids Health Diseases, 2008; 7: 22.

Kalhan A and Rees A. A potential role for monoclonal antibodies in clinical lipidology: can we look beyond statins? Current Opinion in Lipidology, 2013; 24(5): 457–458.

22. B. High-dose statin use has been associated with an increased risk of development of diabetes. The use of corticosteroids is associated with increased insulin resistance, decreased glucose uptake in muscle, and increased gluconeogenesis. Nicotinic acid use has been linked with worsening of glycaemic control, secondary to increased gluconeogenesis. Protease inhibitors that are used as part of anti-retroviral therapy have been shown to induce insulin resistance by inhibition of GLUT4 transporter. Atypical antipsychotic, such as olanzapine and clozapine have been associated with increased risk of diabetes.

Carter A, Gomes T, Camacho X, et al. Risk of incident diabetes among patients treated with statins: population based study. British Medical Journal, 2013; 346: f2610.

Dagogo-Jack S. HIV therapy and diabetes risk. Diabetes care, 2008; 31(6): 1267–1268.

Shen L, Shah B, Reyes E, et al. Role of diuretics, β blockers, and statins in increasing the risk of diabetes in patients with impaired glucose tolerance: reanalysis of data from the NAVIGATOR study. British Medical Journal, 2013; 347: f6745.

23. E. According to NICE guidelines, GLP1 analogue therapy can be considered if the glycaemic control remains suboptimal, despite the use of one or two oral hypoglycaemic agents (metformin, sulfonylureas, glitazones) and:

- The patient has a BMI of 35 kg/m² or over, and has weight-related medical or psychological problems. Or
- The patient has a BMI of <35 kg/m² and insulin would be unacceptable for occupational reasons or weight loss would be beneficial considering significant obesity related co-morbidities.

According to NICE guidelines, the treatment with GLP-1 analogues need to be continued only if there is HbA$_{1c}$ drop of ≥1% and a weight loss of ≥3% 6 months after starting the therapy.

Exenatide therapy needs to be avoided if the eGFR < 30 mL/minute/1.73 m2, while the extended release exenatide and liraglutide need to be avoided if the eGFR < 60 mL/minute/1.73 m².

The main side effects of GLP-1 analogue therapy are gastrointestinal disturbance, including nausea and vomiting, diarrhoea, and abdominal pain. These agents are believed to increase pancreatic duct cell proliferation, leading to low grade pancreatic inflammation and increased pancreatic enzyme levels. The previously mentioned changes can potentially predispose to development of pancreatic cancer, although this needs to be clarified by further research and trials.

NICE. Type 2 diabetes: the management of type 2 diabetes. Guideline CG87. NICE, 2009.

24. E. SGLT-2 inhibitor use is associated with the increased risk of development of urinary tract and genital infections. As these agents promote diuresis, a modest drop in blood pressure may be observed. Dapagliflozin should not be used:

- Along with a loop diuretic.
- In elderly patients.
- If eGFR is <60 mL/minute/1.73 m².
- Along with pioglitazone.
- Presence of diabetic ketoacidosis.

There is no increased risk of hypoglycaemia when these agents are used as monotherapy, although there is an increased risk of hypoglycaemic episodes if used in combination with a sulfonylurea or insulin.

Clar C, Gill A, Court R, et al. Systematic review of SGLT2 receptor inhibitors in dual or triple therapy in type 2 diabetes. British Medical Journal, 2012; 2: e00136.

25. B. Liver and kidneys are the primary organs participating in the process of gluconeogenesis in human beings.

Gerich J, Meyer C, Woerle H, et al. Renal gluconeogenesis: its importance in human glucose homeostasis. Diabetes Care, 2001; 24(2): 382–391.

26. E. Type 2 diabetes is associated with whole spectrum of liver diseases, including abnormal liver function tests, non-alcoholic hepatosteatosis, cirrhosis, and hepatocellular carcinoma. According to the Verona diabetes study, cirrhosis was the fourth leading cause of death in patients with diabetes. Diabetes is also emerging as one of the commonest aetiology of patients otherwise labelled as cryptogenic cirrhosis. Patients with poorly-controlled diabetes characteristically have elevated triglycerides, low HDL cholesterol, elevated LDL-cholesterol levels, with varying degrees of insulin resistance. There is increased lipolysis resulting in elevated levels of free fatty acids and overloading of hepatic mitochondrial β-oxidation system. Free fatty acids induce the production of oxygen free radicals and generation of pro-inflammatory cytokines, such as TNF-α, and interleukin-1 and 6 leading to cellular damage.

Tolman K, Fonesca V, Dalpiaz A, et al. Spectrum of liver disease in type 2 diabetes and management of patients with diabetes and liver disease. Diabetes Care, 2007; 30(3): 734–743.

27. B. Haemochromatosis (bronze diabetes) is a hereditary (*HFE/SCL11A3/HAMP* gene mutations) or acquired (e.g. secondary to repeated blood transfusions) disorder, which leads to excessive iron accumulation in various tissues and organs, such as pancreas, liver, heart, and joints. Patients can present with non-specific symptoms such as fatigue and malaise, low libido, arthritis, late onset diabetes, liver disorders, bronzed skin, and cardiomyopathy.

Patients with haemochromatosis have an increased transferrin saturation (normal <30%), with elevated ferritin levels (it may be normal in early disease). Liver biopsy and genetic tests are helpful to establish the diagnosis.

Capell P. Case study: haemochromatosis in type 2 diabetes. Clinical Diabetes, 2004; 22(2): 101–102.

Utzschneider K and Kowdley K. Hereditary haemochromotosis and diabetes mellitus: Implications for clinical practice. Nature Reviews Endocrinology, 2010; 6(1): 26–33.

28. A. According to NICE guidelines for the management of diabetes in pregnancy (clinical guideline 63), the following have been shown as independent risk factors for development of gestational diabetes:

1. Body mass index >30 kg/m².
2. Family history of diabetes (first degree relatives).

3. Previous gestational diabetes.
4. Previous macrosomic baby (weighing >4.5 kg).
5. South East Asian/Black Caribbean or Middle Eastern ethnic origin.

Data from NICE guidelines (CG63) Diabetes in pregnancy: Management of diabetes and its complications from pre-conception to the postnatal period. Published March 2008.

NICE. Diabetes in pregnancy: management of diabetes and its complications from pre-conception to the postnatal period. Guideline CG63. NICE, 2008.

29. C. According to NICE guidelines for the management of diabetes in pregnancy (CG63), pre-conception care and assessment of patients with diabetes should include:

- Folic acid (5 mg/day) supplement till week 12 of pregnancy.
- Self-monitoring of blood glucose.
- Ketone testing strips to women with type 1 DM.
- Monthly HbA_{1c}.
- Retinal assessment if not done in the previous 1 year.
- Renal assessment and consideration for referral to renal physician if eGFR <45 mL/minute/1.73 m^2.
- Advice to avoid pregnancy if HbA_{1c} >10%.

Data from NICE guidelines (CG63) Diabetes in pregnancy: Management of diabetes and its complications from pre-conception to the postnatal period. Published March 2008.

NICE. Diabetes in pregnancy: management of diabetes and its complications from pre-conception to the postnatal period. Guideline CG63. NICE, 2008.

30. B. There is a 1.5–2-fold risk of developing major congenital malformations in children born to mothers with type 1 DM compared with the non-diabetic population. The commonest congenital malformations include cardiac, renal, and neural tube defects. There is no conclusive evidence of differences in perinatal mortality and congenital malformation risk in the offspring of women with type 1 or type 2 DM.

Macintosh M, Fleming K, Baily J, et al. Perinatal mortality and congenital anomalies in babies of women with type 1 or type 2 diabetes in England, Wales, and Northern Ireland: population based study. British Medical Journal, 2006; 333: 177.

31. A. The following factors have been linked with poor pregnancy outcome (miscarriage, increased risk of foetal congenital anomalies, perinatal mortality) in a patient with diabetes:

- Maternal social deprivation.
- Unplanned pregnancy.
- Lack of preconception folic acid.
- Smoking.
- Suboptimal preconception diabetes control.
- Antenatal evidence of foetal growth restriction.
- Pre-existing diabetes complications.

NICE. Diabetes in pregnancy: management of diabetes and its complications from pre-conception to the postnatal period. Guideline CG63. NICE, 2008.

32. D. According to NICE guidelines for the management of diabetes in pregnancy:

- Women with diabetes are advised to measure fasting and 1-hour post-prandial blood glucose levels during pregnancy.

- Aim for a fasting blood glucose level 3.5–5.9 mmol/L and a 1-hour post-prandial glucose level < 7.8 mmol/L.
- HbA$_{1c}$ should not be measured routinely in the second and third trimester.
- Individualized targets for monitoring need to be agreed.

Data from NICE guidelines (CG63) Diabetes in pregnancy: Management of diabetes and its complications from pre-conception to the postnatal period. Published March 2008.

NICE. Diabetes in pregnancy: management of diabetes and its complications from pre-conception to the postnatal period. Guideline CG63. NICE, 2008.

33. C. According to NICE guidelines (CG63), there is strong evidence of safety and effectiveness of metformin and glibenclamide therapy during pregnancy. Isophane insulin is a safe long-acting insulin option to be used in women with diabetes during antenatal period. There is no evidence of adverse foetal outcome with the use of short-acting insulin analogues aspart and lispro in antenatal period. Statin and ACE inhibitor therapy need to be stopped during antenatal period.

Data from NICE guidelines (CG63) Diabetes in pregnancy: Management of diabetes and its complications from pre-conception to the postnatal period. Published March 2008.

NICE. Diabetes in pregnancy: management of diabetes and its complications from pre-conception to the postnatal period. Guideline CG63. NICE, 2008.

34. E. There is a 4-fold increased perinatal mortality in children born to mothers with diabetes, compared with the non-diabetic population. There is no conclusive evidence of differences in perinatal mortality and congenital malformation risk in the offspring of women with type 1 or type 2 DM.

Macintosh M, Fleming K, Baily J, et al. Perinatal mortality and congenital anomalies in babies of women with type 1 or type 2 diabetes in England, Wales, and Northern Ireland: population based study. British Medical Journal 2006; 333: 177.

35. A. Table 6.3 compares the diagnostic criteria for gestational diabetes (GDM) based on 75-g oral glucose tolerance test.

Table 6.3 WHO and IADPSG criteria for diagnosis of GDM

	IADPSG	WHO/NICE
Fasting	>5.1 mmol/L	>7.0 mmol/L
1 hour	>10 mmol/L	–
2 hour	>8.5 mmol/L	>7.8 mmol/L

Data from World Health Organization, Diagnostic Criteria and Classification of Hyperglycaemia First Detected in Pregnancy, 2013; and International Association of Diabetes and Pregnancy Study Groups Recommendations on the Diagnosis and Classification of Hyperglycemia in Pregnancy. Diabetes Care March 2010; 33 (3): 676–682.

The results from the multinational Hyperglycaemia and Pregnancy Outcome (HAPO) study, comprising 23,000 subjects showed a linear relationship between maternal fasting blood glucose and OGTT at 1 and 2 hours with birthweight above the 90th percentile. It also demonstrated a linear relationship between infantile adiposity and maternal glucose levels. Based on application of the IADPSG criteria, about 16% of pregnant women will be diagnosed with gestational diabetes, compared with about 3.5%, based on current practice leading to huge implications on resources. On the other hand, most of these women can be managed by diet and lifestyle modification with insulin treatment required in only 10–15% of these women. Gestational diabetes is also linked with an increased risk of developing obesity in later life, making it even more crucial to identify and manage it more pro-actively compared with the current practice.

International Association of Diabetes and Pregnancy Study Groups Recommendations on the Diagnosis and Classification of Hyperglycemia in Pregnancy. Diabetes Care, 2010; 33(3): 676–682.

36. B. HbA$_{1c}$ measurement is the standard laboratory test for the assessment of glycaemic control. Clinical conditions that affect haemoglobin lifespan and haemoglobinopathies can impact reliability of HbA$_{1c}$ results (falsely low readings). In contrast, falsely-elevated HbA$_{1c}$ values can be seen in uraemia (carbamoylated Hb) or in the presence of Hb F.

This man had suboptimal glycaemic control as reflected by his elevated home blood sugar readings, although his HbA$_{1c}$ is low (falsely low due to underlying sickle cell disease). As a result, his insulin dose needs to be increased to improve glycaemic control.

In patients with haemoglobinopathies, measurement of fructosamine may provide a better assessment of glycaemic control compared with HbA$_{1c}$. Fructosamine measurement is dependent on serum protein glycation and remains unaffected by the presence of haemoglobinopathies. In contrast to HbA$_{1c}$, fructosamine measurement provides assessment regarding blood glucose levels during preceding 2–3 weeks only.

Kilpatrick E and Winocour P. ABCD position statement on haemoglobin A1c for diagnosis of diabetes. Practical Diabetes International, 2010; 27(6): 306–310.

37. A. The presence of haemoglobinopathy, haemolytic anaemia, renal impairment, and pregnancy may be associated with a false negative HbA1c results. Doxazosin has no known impact on HbA1c values.

Kilpatrick E and Winocour P. ABCD position statement on haemoglobin A1c for diagnosis of diabetes. Practical Diabetes International, 2010; 27(6): 306–310.

38. A. Fibrates reduce triglyceride levels by increasing lipoprotein lipase activity. These are more efficacious than statins to reduce triglyceride levels and increasing HDL-cholesterol, although less effective in lowering LDL-cholesterol compared with the statins. In type 2 DM, statins are generally employed as the first-line agent to manage dyslipidaemia.

According to the NICE guidelines (CG87 type 2 diabetes):

- Assess possible secondary causes of high serum triglycerides (e.g. poor glycaemic control, hypothyroidism, renal impairment, and liver inflammation) and if any of these causes is identified, manage accordingly.
- In the absence of secondary causes of elevated triglycerides, consider starting fibrates if levels remain > 4.5 mmol/L.
- Statin and fibrate therapy can be combined if the triglyceride levels remain elevated (2.3–4.5 mmol/L) despite statin therapy in high cardiovascular risk patients.

Data from NICE guidelines (CG87) Type 2 diabetes: The management of Type 2 diabetes. May 2009.

NICE . Type 2 diabetes: the management of type 2 diabetes. NICE guideline CG87, 2009.

39. B. Vitamin A is essential to maintain visual acuity, immunological functions, and cellular proliferation. It is present as pro-vitamin carotenoids in plant sources and retinyl palmitate in animal sources. The incidence of vitamin A deficiency has been reported between 5 and 10% after bariatric surgery, according to various reports. Vitamin A deficiency is associated with night blindness, xerophthalmia, and occasionally complete blindness. Night blindness usually manifests as an inability in adjustment to dimmed light and is an early feature of vitamin A deficiency. The production of eye pigment, rhodopsin (which is responsible for sensing low light situations) is impaired in patients with vitamin A deficiency.

40. C. Albuminuria (urinary albumin excretion rate >300 mg/24 hours) is usually measured as a urinary albumin:creatinine ratio. There is marked variability in albumin excretion on a day-to-day basis as a result; according to NICE guidelines a positive test for urine albumin to creatinine ration-eeds to be repeated at least twice more, with a patient deemed to have albuminuria if two of these three tests are positive (raised urine ACR). The presence of albuminuria in this gentleman is an indicator of diabetic nephropathy. Blood pressure control using ACE inhibitors will be the most useful next therapeutic step. ACE inhibitors act by lowering the intraglomerular filtration pressure. In clinical practice, his glycaemic control needs to be improved, with a lowering of his LDL-cholesterol. Albuminuria is also predictive of cardiovascular morbidity and mortality in patients with diabetes.

Basi S, Fesler P, Mimran A, et al. Microalbuminuria in type 2 diabetes and hypertension: a marker, treatment target, or innocent bystander. Diabetes Care, 2008; 31(2): S194–S201.

Diabetic nephropathy, treatment: BMJ Best Practice, http://bestpractice.bmj.com/best-practice/monograph/530.html.

41. A. According to NICE guidelines on the management of overweight and obese adults (NICE CG43), should consider surgery for people with severe obesity if they are:

- Achieved or nearly achieved physiological maturity.
- Under intensive specialist management.
- A BMI of 40 kg/m^2 or more, or a BMI of 35–40kg/m^2 in the presence of other significant disease (e.g. type 2 diabetes, high blood pressure, osteoarthritis, sleep apnoea) that could be improved if they lost weight.
- All appropriate non-surgical measures have failed to achieve or maintain adequate clinically beneficial weight loss for at least 6 months.
- Receiving or will receive intensive specialist management.
- Generally fit for anaesthesia and surgery.
- Committed for long-term follow-up.

Data from NICE guidelines (CG43) Obesity: Guidance on the prevention, identification, assessment and management of overweight and obesity in adults and children. Published in December 2006.

NICE. Obesity: guidance on the prevention, identification, assessment and management of overweight and obesity in adults and children. Guideline 43. NICE, 2006.

42. B. According to NICE guidelines (Technology appraisal 151, issued July 2008) insulin pump therapy should be considered in adults and children >12 years of age with type 1 diabetes if:

- Attempts to reach target HbA$_{1c}$ with multiple insulin injections is leading to disabling hypoglycaemic episodes. Or
- HbA$_{1c}$ levels >8.5%, despite multiple daily insulin injections.

Data from NICE technology appraisals (TA151) Continuous subcutaneous insulin infusion for the treatment of diabetes mellitus. Published in July 2008.

NICE. Continuous subcutaneous insulin infusion for the treatment of diabetes mellitus. Technology appraisal TA151. NICE, 2008.

43. C. The serum osmolality in this patient is 292 mOsmol/kg, despite having low sodium of 106 mmol/L, suggestive of high blood glucose values:

- Serum osmolality: 2 × Na + urea + glucose.
- 292 mOsmol/Kg = 2 × 106 + 30 + glucose.
- 292 mOsmol/kg = 212 + 30 + glucose.
- 292 mosmol/kg = 242 + glucose.
- Glucose = 292 − 242 = 50 mmol/L.

The correct management approach for this patient is to start intravenous fluids and insulin infusion as he is clinically dehydrated with elevated blood glucose levels, with having a translocational hyponatraemia.

Rao LN, Kalhan A, Bolusani H, et al. Translocational hyponatraemia—an important clue to the diagnosis of hyperosmotic hyponatraemia secondary to hyperglycaemic crisis. British Journal of Diabetes & Vascular Disease, 2012; 12(1): 54–56.

44. A. This woman has secondary hypothyroidism in view of her biochemical results of low FT4 and inappropriately low normal TSH. She has presented with sudden onset of headache and nausea, and pituitary apoplexy should be considered as a diagnosis.

Pituitary apoplexy may occur on background of expansion of a pre-existing pituitary adenoma, which may or may not have been diagnosed previously. The features of sudden-onset headache and ophthalmoplegia (3rd, 4th, and 6th nerve palsies) should be alert for the possibility of pituitary apoplexy. The initiation of steroids in these settings may be life-saving. It is a differential diagnosis of angiographically negative subarachnoid haemorrhage.

Rajasekaran S, Vanderpump M, Baldeweg S, et al. UK guidelines for the management of pituitary apoplexy. Pituitary Apoplexy Guidelines Development Group, May 2010. Clinical Endocrinology, 2011; 74: 9–20.

45. D. This man has biochemical features of dehydration (elevated urea levels); his low Na level is most probably due to hypovolaemic hyponatraemia, rather than SIADH. The key point to remember in clinical practice is that the urinary spot sodium test results are influenced by hydration status, as well as medications being taken. In this patient, despite his relative hypovolaemic state, urinary sodium levels are 40 mmol (rather than <10 mmol as expected in a patient with dehydration) due to the concomitant use of diuretic therapy.

Spasovski G, Vanholder R, Allolio B, et al. Clinical practice guidelines on diagnosis and treatment of hyponatraemia. European Journal of Endocrinology, 2014; 170: G1–G47.

46. E. This patient has euvolaemic hypovolaemia and her biochemistry results are consistent with a diagnosis of syndrome of inappropriate antidiuresis. The vasopressin secretion in patients with syndrome of inappropriate antidiuresis is inappropriate as it occurs independently of effective serum osmolality or circulating volume.

In a patient with acute hyponatraemia due to the syndrome of inappropriate diuresis, 3% saline needs to be used in the presence of red flag features, such as encephalopathic seizures (due to low Na), coma, reduced GCS, or severe symptoms.

Spasovski G, Vanholder R, Allolio B, et al. Clinical practice guidelines on diagnosis and treatment of hyponatraemia. European Journal of Endocrinology, 2014; 170: G1–G47.

47. D. The presence of the following clinical and biochemical characteristics should prompt a search for an alternative aetiology for renal impairment in patients with diabetes:

- Duration of type 2 DM <5 years and type 1 DM <10 years.
- Absence of diabetic retinopathy.
- Presence of active sediment in urine.
- Rapid decline in eGFR.
- Refractory hypertension (systemic hypertension although is common).
- Massive albuminuria.
- >30% decline in eGFR within 2–3 months of initiation of ACE inhibitor or ARB therapy.
- Significant haematuria.
- Presence of systemic illness.

National Kidney Foundation.KDOQI Clinical Practice Guideline for Diabetes and CKD: 2012 update. American Journal of Kidney Disease, 2012; 60(5): 850–886.

NICE. Type 2 diabetes: the management of Type 2 diabetes. Guidelines CG87. NICE, 2009.

48. D. Cystatin C measurement may be useful in clinical circumstances where creatinine measurement may not be appropriate such as:

- Patients with liver cirrhosis.
- Morbid obesity.
- Malnourished patients with small muscle mass.
- In the early detection of kidney disease.

Inker L, Schmid C, Tighiouart H, et al. Estimating glomerular filtration rate from serum creatinine and cystatin C. New England Journal of Medicine, 2012; 367: 20–29.

Shlipak M, Matsushita K, Arnlov J, et al. Cystatin C versus creatinine in determining risk based on kidney function. New England Journal of Medicine, 2013; 369: 932–943.

49. B. According to NICE guidelines (CG96), duloxetine is the first line treatment for patients with painful diabetic neuropathy. Duloxetine is contraindicated in following circumstances:

- eGFR <30 mL/minute/1.73 m^2.
- Pregnancy.
- Hepatic impairment.

Oral amitriptyline (at a lower dose) should be offered if duloxetine is contraindicated. If the patient has unsatisfactory pain reduction, despite being at the maximum tolerated dose of the first-line agent, he/she should be offered a switch to or combination with a second-line treatment option, such as pregablin.

Data from NICE clinical guidelines (CG96) Neuropathic pain: the pharmacological management of neuropathic pain in adults in non-specialist settings. Published in March 2010.

NICE. Neuropathic pain: the pharmacological management of neuropathic pain in adults in non-specialist settings. Guidelines CG96. NICE, 2010.

50. A. According to NICE guidelines (CG15), children and young people with type 1 diabetes should be offered screening for:

- Coeliac disease at diagnosis.
- Thyroid disease at diagnosis (and annually thereafter).
- Retinopathy annually from the age of 12 years.
- Microalbuminuria annually from the age of 12 years.
- Blood pressure annually from the age of 12 years.

Data from NICE guidelines (CG15) Diagnosis and management of type 1 diabetes in children, young people and adults. Published in July 2004.

NICE. Diagnosis and management of type 1 diabetes in children, young people and adults. Guidelines CG15. NICE, 2004.

51. D. In a patient who appears to have type 2 diabetes, consider a diagnosis of type 1 diabetes if he/she has:

- Ketonuria.
- Marked weight loss.
- No features of metabolic syndrome.

Similarly, consider a diagnosis of type 2 diabetes/maturity onset diabetes of diabetes in younger adults in the presence of:

- Obesity.
- Family history of diabetes.

South East Asian men are prone to type 2 DM with a comparatively lower BMI, and measurement of waist circumference is considered more accurate in this particular ethnic group.

NICE. Diagnosis and management of type 1 diabetes in children, young people and adults. Guideline CG15. NICE, 2004.

Khunti K, Kumar S, and Brodie J. Diabetes UK and South Asian Health Foundation recommendations on diabetes research priorities for British South Asians. Diabetes UK, 2009.

52. C. According to NICE guidelines (CG87), the benefits and risks of insulin therapy should be discussed with an individual when control of blood glucose is suboptimal (HbA$_{1c}$ > 7.5% or 58 mmol/mol, or a previously agreed higher level) despite him/her being on two or more oral hypoglycaemic agents.

- Human NPH insulin injected at bed-time or bd remains the initial recommended insulin.
- A long-acting insulin analogue (insulin detemir or glargine) can be considered if:
  - the person needs assistance from carer or healthcare professional to inject insulin to reduce the frequency of injections; or
  - patient's lifestyle is restricted by recurrent symptomatic hypoglycaemic episodes; or
  - patient cannot use the device to inject NPH insulin.
- Pre-mixed (biphasic) human insulin bd can be considered especially if HbA1c > 9.0% (75 mmol/mol).

Data from NICE guidelines (CG87) Type 2 diabetes: The management of Type 2 diabetes. May 2009.

NICE. Type 2 diabetes: the management of Type 2 diabetes. Guideline CG87. NICE, 2009.

53. A. A patient with diabetic retinopathy should be referred to ophthalmology if:

- There are features of maculopathy including exudates or retinal thickening within 1 disc diameter of the centre of the fovea or circinate exudates within the macula.
- There are features of preproliferative retinopathy including any venous beading or venous loops, intra-arterial microvascular abnormalities, multiple deep blot haemorrhages.
- Any unexplained drop in visual acuity.

NICE. Type 2 diabetes: the management of Type 2 diabetes. Guideline CG87. NICE, 2009.

INDEX

Note: Questions appear in bold; answers appear in *italics*

Printed and bound by CPI Group (UK) Ltd, Croydon, CR0 4YY